Problem-Based Psychiatry

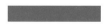

Dr Ben Green

MB ChB MRCPSych
Consultant in Psychological Medicine
Halton General and Winwick Hospitals, UK

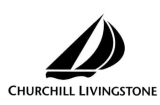

CHURCHILL LIVINGSTONE

NEW YORK, EDINBURGH, LONDON, MADRID, MELBOURNE, SAN FRANCISCO AND TOKYO 1996

CHURCHILL LIVINGSTONE
Medical Division of Pearson Professional Limited

Distributed in the United States of America by Churchill
Livingstone Inc., 650 Avenue of the Americas, New York,
N.Y. 10011, and by associated companies, branches and
representatives throughout the world.

© Pearson Professional Limited 1996

First published 1996

ISBN 0–443–05198–4

British Library Cataloguing in Publication Data
A catalogue record for this book is available from the British
Library

Library of Congress Cataloging in Publication Data
A Catalog record for this book is available from the Library
of Congress

Produced by Longman Singapore Publishers (Pte) Ltd
Printed in Singapore

For Churchill Livingstone

Publisher: Timothy Horne
Project Editor: Jim Killgore
Editor: James Dale
Design Direction: Erik Bigland
Project Controller: Debra Barrie / Nancy Arnott

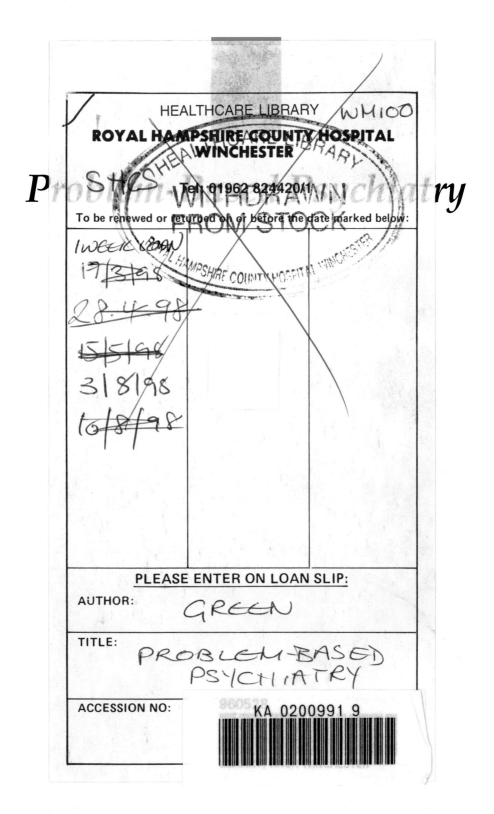

Problem-Based Psychiatry

Dedicated to my wife, Tina, and my son, James

Preface

Medical schools world-wide are having to consider exactly what should go into a medical undergraduate course. The explosion of knowledge and technology has produced a need to reconsider what ideas, facts, attitudes and skills are required of student doctors.

Didactic teaching has long been criticised for its relative inflexibility and the simple fact that much of the knowledge thought to be imparted by such methods is seldom retained for any useful length of time. A more active learning style is therefore required. Problem-based learning (PBL) has come of age now offering a more exciting method of learning and also one where learned knowledge and skills are perhaps more likely to be retained.

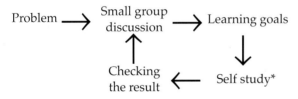

*Each student studies all the learning goals

In several universities, PBL is generally a group endeavour where an initial problem is posed to the group in a tutorial setting. The group discusses the problem and develops its own learning objectives or goals. The group then fragments and the individuals go away to find their own resources to fulfil these goals. Meeting again later in the tutorial group, the problem is revisited and discussed with the benefit of study. New ideas are explored and, hopefully, solutions discovered, although further problems/questions may be identified for further study.

Problem-based Psychiatry presents a series of mini case histories collected on various topics. In the group setting the students would then have to find their own resources to create solutions and explanations. In this book, however, a series of questions usually follows each case together with explanatory answers and suggestions for further reading. The purpose of these explanations is to guide the individual, without group support, through the thinking processes that might underlie a clinician's differential diagnosis or management. At the end of most chapters a section called 'Explorations' offers ideas for further researches that link psychiatry with other basic and clinical sciences.

I hope that *Problem-based Psychiatry* will be found a useful and exciting book which stimulates enthusiasm for the subject. I have enjoyed writing the book and hope that readers will enjoy it too.

BG
1996

Acknowledgements

would like to thank Dr Alex Milosevic of the iverpool Dental School for the images of the ral health consequences of bulimia nervosa; rofessor Nancy Andreasen of the University of owa College of Medicine Mental Health Clinical esearch Center for the MRI images of brain hanges in schizophrenia; Dr Christina Routh, ecturer in Child and Adolescent Psychiatry, Dr David Anderson, Psychiatrist of Old Age, Dr aul Miller, Professor John Copeland and Profesor Greg Wilkinson of the Liverpool University Department of Psychiatry and Dr John Bligh and Mr Philip Evans of the Liverpool Medical Education Unit for their comments and suggestions on sections of the manuscript. I am also grateful to Mr Timothy Horne and Mr Jim Killgore of Churchill Livingstone for their kind help in nurturing this project to its conclusion.

BG
1996

Contents

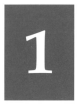

The fundamentals of psychiatry

Psychiatry is a rich and diverse medical specialty concerned with abnormalities of the mind, namely abnormal emotions and thoughts, which may result in abnormal behaviour. Psychiatric illness may have social, psychological and biological causes. The symptoms and signs of mental disorder are known as psychopathology. Doctors analyse a patient's psychopathology using the psychiatric history and the mental state examination.

Contents

Introduction

Psychiatrists use four methods of assessment: the psychiatric history, a mental state examination, a physical examination and relevant medical, social and psychological investigations. Information from these assessment methods is built into a differential diagnosis from which a management plan is formulated. The assessment is a holistic one in that it incorporates physical, social and psychological components. Similarly, treatments for mental illness may involve physical, social and psychological treatments.

- *Physical treatments* may include drugs such as antidepressants and antipsychotics, electroconvulsive therapy (ECT) and, very rarely, psychosurgery.
- *Social treatments* may involve rehousing in special rehabilitation settings, attendance at day hospital or day centres, some family interventions such as giving information and counselling to relatives and socio-legal advice.
- *Psychological treatments* may include one-to-one psychotherapy, group psychotherapy and family therapy. One-to-one psychotherapy is sometimes called interpersonal therapy. There are many different forms, such as psychoanalysis and cognitive therapy.

However, such treatment plans can only be put into place once a diagnosis is made. Before a doctor can make a diagnosis, he or she must first recognise the symptoms and signs of mental illness. Such symptoms and signs are referred to as *psychopathology*.

CASE HISTORY 1

A 24-year-old man is brought to casualty by the police after picking a fight with a taxi driver. He paces up and down restlessly and talks non-stop about an alien space craft from Betelgeuse which is transmitting thoughts into his head. His speech is very difficult to understand. From his appearance it looks as if he has not changed or washed in several weeks.

CASE HISTORY 2

A 72-year-old lady is seen by her family doctor. She complains of not being able to sleep because of 'the people upstairs'. They keep her awake all night with their conversations about her. Sometimes they sing rude limericks about her virginity. The family doctor protests that she lives on the top floor of a block of flats and so there is nobody living above her. However, the old lady is adamant: 'they must be living in the roof space then. I hear them all day long.'

CASE HISTORY 3

A 20-year-old man goes to see his primary care doctor with feelings of panic and anxiety that have come on since the death of his mother 4 weeks before. He is finding it difficult to concentrate on his work and is crying most days.

CASE HISTORY 4

A 70-year-old man is reluctantly brought to the surgery by his wife. He denies that there is anything wrong, but when alone with the doctor she says that his memory is rapidly failing him and recently he has been doing 'odd things' like putting his shoes in the fridge and wearing his vest outside his shirt.

The psychiatric assessment

The four cases above demonstrate that mental illness can occur at any age and that it can have a rich variety of presentations. Making a full assessment helps make sense of these different presentations and helps psychiatrists avoid dangerous diagnostic mistakes such as missing treatable organic disease (like hypothyroidism) and preventing suicide (by assessing whether there are any suicidal fantasies or plans).

The psychiatrist draws the information from this assessment together into a *formulation* which includes a summary, a *differential diagnosis* and a *management plan*. The differential diagnosis depends upon the psychiatrist being aware of how different psychiatric illnesses are classified. The most important or likely diagnoses are considered first and are usually followed by a brief summary of evidence for and against each diagnosis. The differential diagnosis should cover any possible organic causes of symptoms together with the contribution that the patient's personality makes.

Before we go any further, we need to explore some of the range of symptoms and signs that occur in everyday psychiatry.

Psychopathology

Abnormal moods

Affect is our emotional state at any one time. *Mood* is our prevailing emotional state over time. Generally people's mood does vary according to events. Welcome events, like passing exams or getting promotion, make us feel happy. Untoward events, like sudden bereavement or failure, make us feel sad. On the whole, our mood is fairly constant, normal and *euthymic. Dysthymia* suggests an abnormality of mood. Abnormal mood is usually very different from normal in severity and persistence and may be low (*depression*) or high (*mania* or *hypomania*, a lesser form).

Depression is associated with pervasive feelings of sadness. Bouts or crying or feeling like crying may be frequent. Thoughts are usually gloomy. Depressed people think badly of themselves and the future. Usually enjoyable activities are no longer of interest or enjoyment (*anhedonia*). Concentration on tasks, such as reading, is difficult leading to poor function at work or home. Thoughts themselves may seem slowed down and the depressed person may even move less (*psychomotor retardation*), to such an extent that they may become stuporose. Important symptoms associated with depression are the so-called *biological features of depression* which usually include:

- insomnia (particularly intermittent waking through the night and waking earlier in the morning and being unable to return to sleep)
- anorexia (a reduction in the desire for food and subsequently reduced food intake)
- weight loss

- diurnal mood variation (usually a predictable variation in mood through the day, e.g. feeling low and slowed down in the morning and brightening towards the evening)
- reduced sex drive (reduced sexual appetite or libido)
- constipation.

Feelings that life is not worth living or frank thoughts about ending one's life are common amongst depressed people and should be asked about. Asking about these thoughts does not provoke suicidal thoughts or acts, but may enable the patient to express some difficult ideas, feel understood and ultimately may help prevent suicide.

Mania (or its lesser form hypomania) is usually associated with an expansive mood or elation. In contrast to the depressive's gloom the manic patient's thoughts and feelings correspond with the notion that everything is just wonderful. Instead of being psychomotor retarded as in depression, the manic patient's thoughts seem to race along and their activity may be greater than normal, even frantic. The rapid pace of thoughts may lead to fast speech (*pressure of speech*) and a rapid flow of connected ideas (*flight of ideas*), usually on a grand scale. The manic may have grandiose plans based on an overvaluation of their own potential. Their judgement is affected and they may feel that they are inordinately wealthy or just about to make a million from some unlikely scheme.

This may lead to *overspending* or other errors of judgement in work or business. The elated mood of such patients can be enjoyable for those around them, but the elation may be associated with irritability. When confronted the disinhibited manic patient may become violent. Mood swings are possible and the happy mood may easily switch into a depressed one. Suicidal feelings may occur.

Insomnia is nearly always present and patients may give a history of intense activity at times when they would normally be asleep, e.g. spring cleaning the entire house at 3 a.m.

Abnormal thoughts

Through the course of a normal day a variety of thoughts and fantasies pass through the average person's mind. Sometimes people are *preoccupied* by certain thoughts, and this may be relevant and understandable, e.g. often thinking about a driving test in the days beforehand. Occasionally some thoughts may enter a person's mind unbidden and, although the person knows that these thoughts of theirs are irrational or nonsensical, the thoughts keep on recurring no matter how hard they try to resist them. Such thoughts are *obsessions*. An example might be a vicar who has a repeated *intrusive thought* that someone has urinated in the holy water in the church font. Sometimes a person may dwell on an unusual topic to a morbid degree, e.g. a sweet shop owner who campaigns that chocolate should be recommended by doctors for its mood enhancing properties. Such an thought would be an *overvalued idea*. It is sometimes difficult to fault the detail of an overvalued idea. After all, as in the example, chocolate does have some mood enhancing properties, but is the idea worth campaigning about to the exclusion of other pursuits? Where a person holds a belief that is manifestly untrue, is not culturally accepted, and holds it with an intensity that cannot be argued against, then this is a *delusion*. A delusion is an example of a severe or *psychotic* symptom. The presence of a delusion suggests a major or *psychotic* illness.

Delusions can take different forms. In severe depressive illness patients may have delusions of poverty (e.g. that they have no money when they are in fact comfortably off), *hypochondriacal delusions* (e.g. that they have terminal cancer when there is no evidence for this at all), delusions of infestation (e.g. that they are infested with insects after a guilty sexual liaison), or sometimes so-called *nihilistic* delusions, such that they may say 'I have no head' or 'I have no heart'.

In mania, delusions may be expansive or *grandiose*, e.g. 'I am related to the King and he will send me a million pounds next week.'

Sometimes delusions, as in schizophrenia, may be bizarre, e.g. 'I was born from a Vulcan father and an Andromedan mother who gave birth to me in a McDonalds restaurant last week.'

In paranoid, or persecutory, schizophrenia there may be *delusions of reference* in which the patient is certain that a variety of cues in the environment are personally related to them, e.g. a patient called Brian Murray Walker who feels that all BMW advertisements refer specially to him or another patient who feels that the television newscaster is giving him coded messages when he blinks on screen.

Abnormal experiences

Some experiences may be rare or unusual, others may be so unusual as to suggest a major or psychotic illness. *Depersonalisation* is an example of an experience that is not everyday, but may occasionally be experienced in 'normal' people. It is the sense that something has changed in the perception of the self, a feeling of unreality which may be quite unpleasant. Depersonalisation may occur in those who are tired or unwell. *Derealisation* is a related phenomenon where one feels that the world around (rather than the self) has become unreal. A variant of this is the change in the experience of time — the feeling of *déjà vu* where the person feels that they have experienced an exactly similar event before. *Jamais vu* occurs when the person feels that they have never experienced a familiar event before. Such experiences may occur in anyone given the setting of tiredness or physical ill health but may also occur in any psychiatric illness. They may be suggestive of temporal lobe epilepsy.

We experience the world through our senses. An experience is usually the same thing as a perception. In other words, our perception of reality usually accords with reality, i.e. we see what is actually there. We perceive real stimuli. When we misperceive real stimuli this may be an example of an *illusion*. In an illusion our brain misinterprets a real object. The misinterpretation may be because of an extreme affect, e.g. fear, or some problem in processing the information, e.g. tiredness or disorientation due, say, to an infectious illness. An example of an illusion is the scene in Disney's *Snow White* where the princess runs through the dark forest seconds after nearly being attacked by the huntsman and his knife. In her fright the princess misperceives the hollows in the trees around her as gaping eyes and mouths and the trees' branches as claw-like hands. This, then, is a visual illusion. Illusions may also occur in other sensory systems.

Hallucinations are sensory perceptions where there is no stimulus, i.e. no object. Hallucinations can occur in any sensory system too. An auditory hallucination might be hearing a voice talking to you when there is nobody or nothing around to produce that voice. If you look again at Case history 2 you may agree that the patient here might be hallucinating.

Hallucinations are real in quality — just as real as any voice or any real-life image. They are also experienced in *external space*, that is to say they are not experienced as being inside the patient's head.

Hallucinations may occasionally occur in 'normal' people when they are tired or physically unwell. *Hypnagogic* hallucinations are hallucinations occurring on the edge of falling asleep, such as hearing one's name called when there is nobody there. Hallucinations on waking are called *hypnopompic* hallucinations. Occasionally people who have been bereaved may transiently hear or see the lost one. These are known as *pseudohallucinations of mourning*. All these may occur rarely and episodically in 'normal' people. However, persistent hallucinations outside these rare circumstances are psychotic symptoms and suggestive of psychotic illness.

Severe depressive illness may be associated with derogatory auditory hallucinations such as voices telling the patient they smell, are guilty or doomed. These hallucinations are mood congruent. In mania, auditory hallucinations may correspond to the expansive mood and praise the patient. Visual hallucinations are less common than auditory ones and suggest the possibility of organic factors such as brain lesions or drug side-effects. Olfactory hallucinations are rare and may suggest a frontal lobe tumour. Somatic hallucinations occasionally occur with some drugs of abuse and in delirium tremens, but may occur in schizophrenia. Auditory hallucinations may be of a voice or voices talking to the patient (*second person auditory hallucinations*) or may be voices talking about the patient, say in a discussion amongst themselves (*third person auditory hallucinations*). Third person hallucinations are suggestive of schizophrenia.

Still more unusual experiences involve the nature of thought itself. In *thought interference* the patient may feel that their thoughts are being tampered with. Normally we feel as if we 'own' our thoughts. In some psychotic illnesses people may feel as if their thoughts are not their own. They may feel that thoughts have been put into their head (*thought insertion* as in Case history 1), or taken out of their head (*thought withdrawal*) or feel that their thoughts are simultaneously known by others (*thought broadcasting*).

Thought interference is an example of a *passivity phenomenon* where the patient feels that the ownership of thoughts, feelings or actions is in doubt. Other passivity phenomena may include *made feelings*, e.g. 'this isn't my happiness, it's someone else's' or *made actions*, e.g. 'my leg can move, but it isn't me moving it'.

Passivity phenomena are suggestive of schizophrenia.

Abnormal forms of thought

You can describe thought in terms of its *content*, i.e. what it is about, or in terms of its *form*, i.e. how it is shaped. In mania there may be a flood of thoughts, rapidly spilling out of the mind and expressed in a pressure of speech. The form of these thoughts may be so-called *flight of ideas* in which there are a large number of ideas but where each idea is linked one to another by subject matter, by puns or sounds:

> *I see you're wearing sandals, Third World shoes, sandy shoes, Road to Damascus shoes, conversion shoes, brilliant light shoes, on your knees in front of the Spirit, the Spirit inside the bottle, the genial genie genius of my soul.*

Although such speech may seem unintelligible at first, when analysed later each item can be linked to another. In the above example the speaker is reminded of St.Paul's conversion on the road to Damascus by the sandals that someone else is wearing.

When the associations between the items of speech are lost (*loosening of associations*), this may represent *thought disorder*, which is seen in schizophrenia and other states. Here it is much less easy to spot an association between thoughts:

> *on the albigisty of Kama sura I swear that the lazy dog leapt twice and danced on the afternoon Sun, buthga, buthga, buthagee, where in fact the News at Ten is never at two. Have you a cigarette he asks, she asks. Never.*

The above example contains some examples of *neologisms* or new words, such as 'albigisty'. Such neologisms may occur in schizophrenic speech. Similarly, more familiar words may be used inappropriately.

Abnormal movements

Since psychological symptoms and treatments often involve the central nervous system, abnormal movements may be associated with a mental disorder. They may be idiopathic, symptomatic of the illness, a side-effect of drug treatment or signify a neurological disease such as neurosyphilis or Huntington's chorea.

Tics, occasional rhythmic involuntary movements such as eye blinking or occasionally vocalisations, may be common in childhood and of little prognostic significance. They tend to diminish of their own accord, but often worsen if attention is drawn to them or the patient is made to feel anxious. Rarely tics may be progressive and disabling as in *Gilles de la Tourette's* syndrome, which is sometimes associated with obscene vocal tics (*coprolalia*).

Mannerisms are repeated voluntary movements that are idiosyncratic to the point of oddness, e.g. saluting twice before entering a room. *Posturing* may be prolonged and stereotyped or manneristic. Posturing is sometimes seen in schizophrenic illnesses. *Catatonia* in its most severe form involves the patient becoming mute, stuporose and prone to abnormal preservation of postures. In this catatonic state patients' limbs may be moved by observers and the resulting posture preserved for hours. *Akathisia*, *tardive dyskinesia* and *Parkinsonism* are often seen in patients taking psychiatric medications (see chapter 15, 'Physical treatments'). Akathisia is a drug-induced restlessness which may be described by the patient or observed as agitated fidgeting in a chair or aimless pacing about the room. Tardive dyskinesia is a basal ganglia movement disorder manifesting as a combination of involuntary rhythmic movements of any of the following: lips, tongue, face, arms, hands, legs, feet or trunk. Sometimes it may be observed as choreo-athetoid movements. Tardive dyskinesia is thought to be a late side-effect of neuroleptic drugs. Parkinsonism may be an early side-effect of such drugs and may manifest with classical Parkinsonian features such as mask-like features, pill-rolling tremor and bradykinesia.

Interview skills

The psychiatric history is lengthier and more detailed than in other fields of medicine. It covers aspects of personality, psychiatric illness and personal biography as well as a detailed medical history. To get this information the psychiatrist may interview the patient and an informant such as a relative, friend or other close acquaintance (but only with the patient's consent).

Since the history seeks to include sensitive information about past events and feelings past and present, the style is different from a conventional medical history. When you start taking psychiatric histories, the interview may extend to 90 minutes. With practice you will be able to gather the most relevant information more quickly, but it is important to remember that patients need time and to feel that their doctor is genuinely interested if they are to disclose personal details. Accordingly, psychiatric interviews sometimes appear less controlled by the doctor, who uses more open questions and empathic statements. Open questions are often used at the beginning of a section of questions on, say, family history, and will allow the patient to talk about important aspects as they see them, e.g. 'Can you begin by telling me about your family?' To regain control of the interview or gather specific information closed questions need to be used, e.g. 'what age was your father when he died?' or 'Which drugs helped you in the past?' or 'Do you ever feel like harming yourself?'

Statements, if used carefully, show that you understand what the patient is talking about from their point of view. Psychotic experiences are distressing ones, often associated with fear. Acknowledging this in some way would make a patient think that their doctor knew something about the symptoms and also understood how they really felt. Being understood is a positive experience for anyone and is reassuring.

CASE HISTORY 5

Alan was talking to the doctor. Tears of anxiety and fear came to his eyes when he was describing the voices that afflicted him. A strong male voice threatened him night and day, telling him he was about to be killed. 'That must be very frightening,' said his doctor. Alan looked up and nodded vigorously.

Verbal and non-verbal cues can also show interest. Nodding your head or making occasional noises such as 'uh-huh' can be encouraging if they are not overdone. Remaining silent for a short time or pausing before making further statements or questions may allow the patient space to disclose something else. Sometimes inexperienced doctors feel that silence is a bad or uncomfortable thing and that it must be filled with some statement. However, the statements may be ill-thought out, e.g. false reassurance such as 'I'm sure everything will be all right' can appear inappropriate or just plain wrong. In such cases the doctor is often trying to reassure him- or herself rather than the patient.

How will you cope with any expressions of emotion that the patient makes? What if they cry? What if they are irritable, angry or shout? What if they will not sit still long enough? A useful technique is to *reflect* the emotion back — acknowledge that you have noticed their distress or their anger, perhaps even ask about it. Sometimes people cry just before they say something really important, so do not shut them up: support them and let them speak. Anger may precede violence, especially if the patient is afraid. Whatever you do, try and stay calm. Saying that you have noticed how angry they are and asking them to talk about it may defuse the anger. Try not to appear threatening yourself. If an attack seems likely call for help or leave the room. Before you interview potentially dangerous patients always make sure that you have checked with staff who know the patient and that you interview the patient in a known safe place, with ready back up in case of trouble. Having said this, violence is uncommon, and most patients you interview will probably be very cooperative.

People are sensitive to the moods of those they are speaking to. Just as the doctor can pick up on cues as to the patient's mood, the patient can pick up on whether their doctor is anxious, tired and ill-disposed towards them. It is important, therefore, to think about how you appear to the patient and to concentrate on the patient you are with in the here and now. Plenty of agencies will try to distort the doctor-patient relationship for their own ends. It is important not to be distracted from this central relationship by time considerations or matters of politics such as budgetary and rationing decisions. Every communication with the patient is special.

The psychiatric history

Think how you might begin a long interview with someone. What would you do? How would you greet the person? How would you introduce yourself? Would you say how long the interview was going to take? Perhaps you might explain why you want to talk at all. Would you reassure the person about confidentiality?

Demographic details

You can begin the history proper by taking demographic details — age, marital status, employment status and, if in hospital, whether they are there voluntarily or are detained compulsorily. The patient's age, marital and employment status all have a bearing on diagnosis and management. Different mental illnesses have different ages of onset. Schizophrenia has its main onset in the third decade, dementia in the seventh and subsequent decades. The unemployed are more likely to suffer from depression and suicides are more common in the unmarried, widowed and divorced.

Presenting complaint

The presenting complaint is usually a brief list of the major problems as explained by the patient, e.g. 'hearing voices all the time' or 'drinking too much'.

History of presenting complaint

The history of presenting complaint (HPC) records further details. In terms of details it is sometimes useful to compare psychological pain (such as depression) with physical pain. Surgeons will inquire as to the severity of the pain, its character, its onset, whether it is persistent or not and whether it is getting better or is aggravated by any particular thing. Similarly, in a case of depression, psychiatrists are interested in how it started: did it start suddenly or gradually? Did anything happen to bring on the depression such as a bereavement or a loss of job, or was the onset insidious and gradual? Is the pain getting worse or better? Can it be made better by visitors or entertainment or is it persistent? Psychiatrists would ask at this time about the so-called biological features of depression as described above. The HPC would also focus on how severe the patient felt the depression was — is the patient crying every day or only once a week? It is sometimes appropriate to ask at this point whether the patient feels that life is not worth living and, if not, then has the depressed patient thought about harming themselves and do they have any definite plans? Students are often unsure about how to ask about suicidal feelings. Usually psychiatrists ask a hierarchy of questions to elicit these feelings, for an example see Case history 6.

If a patient complained of hearing voices, an attempt would be made to discern exactly what these voices were like — were they hallucinations or illusions, for instance. If the doctor suspected schizophrenia, it would be appropriate in the HPC to ask for other features of schizophrenia, just as in a case of suspected appendicitis the surgeon would ask about fever and features of urinary tract infection to aid in making his or her differential diagnosis.

CASE HISTORY 6

Adam seemed very low to the interviewing doctor. He had biological features of depression such as early morning wakening, diurnal mood variation and poor appetite. He said that he was crying most days but was almost ashamed to tell the doctor. 'Makes me feel like a baby,' he said. He had felt this way for 2 months ever since he had lost his job and his girlfriend.

'It sounds as if things feel really bad,' said the doctor. Adam grunted, but avoided the doctor's gaze. 'Have you ever felt that life wasn't worth living at all?' Adam nodded slowly. 'That you'd rather it was all over?' Another nod. 'Have you thought about doing anything about that?'

'I keep thinking about it. Not all the time, I just get this picture suddenly, for a few seconds, of me running my car into a motorway bridge.'

'Would you do anything like that? Or anything else to harm yourself?'

'No,' said Adam. 'I push the thought out of my head. If I did anything like that it would be too hurtful for my friends and my Mum.'

Past psychiatric history

A useful probe at the beginning of this section might be 'Have you ever felt like this before?' or 'Have you ever seen a psychiatrist before?' In the past psychiatric history the doctor is trying to build up a picture of how the illness has affected the patient in the past. The psychiatrist wishes to learn when the illness began and how many episodes there have been, who treated these illnesses and how successful treatment was — in particular which treatments were most useful. Bear in mind though that not all psychiatric illness presents to psychiatrists or even to doctors at all, so that the true onset of an illness may be a long time before the psychiatrist is called in. Try and get a picture of how many episodes of illness there have been. How long did each episode last? And between episodes how well was the patient? Were they able to resume their work or care for their family as usual? Some illnesses impair function even between acute episodes. For any hospital admission you need to know which hospital it was (useful for getting past notes), which consultant, how long the admission was for and whether they were detained formally or informally (voluntarily). Record any use of antipsychotics, antidepressants, benzodiazepines and electroconvulsive therapy (ECT).

Past medical history

The past medical history is particularly relevant because various physical illnesses may mimic mental illness: hypothyroidism may present with depression, serum B_{12} deficiency may present with dementia and hyperthyroidism may present with persecutory ideas. Drugs that are used to treat physical illnesses may cause psychiatric presentations: digoxin may cause confusion and ranitidine may cause depression. The psychiatrist is, therefore, interested in current and past physical problems including major operations, e.g. orchidectomy and hysterectomy may be complicated by depression and low esteem, and past head trauma may provoke epileptic phenomena.

Family history

The family history should include details of parents, siblings and sometimes children. You should probe for occurrences of mental illness and suicide in any other relatives. It sometimes helps to record the family history in a family tree diagram with notes about each family member on the tree (Fig. 1.1). You should not be purely interested in the psychiatric history of other family members, although it is very relevant because certain psychiatric illnesses cluster in families. This is an opportunity to discuss the patient's feelings about parents, brothers and sisters (siblings). It is of great value to know, for instance, that a patient has never felt able to burden their mother with their anxieties because the mother had suffered with depression as well, or that the father was an argumentative man with an alcohol problem who used to beat his wife (the patient's mother). The family has been found to be important in the aetiology of personality difficulties, anorexia nervosa, bulimia nervosa and the prognosis of schizophrenia. Patients with schizophrenia are more likely to relapse in families where there is a high level of expressed emotion (hostility, over-

involvement by other members and high levels of face to face contact).

Personal history

In order to understand someone better it is often important to know what has happened to them in the past. The personal history seeks to build up a biography from birth to the present day. Early events in a person's life can fundamentally change the course their life takes. Early separation can colour just how secure people are in all their subsequent relationships. Early perinatal brain damage can affect IQ or lead to disabling epilepsy. There are hypotheses linking perinatal damage, febrile convulsions and adult psychotic illnesses. It is, therefore, important to know details as far back as possible. Gather information about the individual's birth — was it a normal full-term vaginal delivery or an induced or instrumental birth. Was there any event, such as time spent in a special care baby unit, that might have affected the maternal-infant relationship (perhaps making it a distant one or even over-close). Is there any evidence for delay in reaching milestones such as the first steps or the first words? Can the person remember any details of what life was like when they were small? Were they hospitalised for any reason? Were their memories happy or not? Did they get on with their siblings?

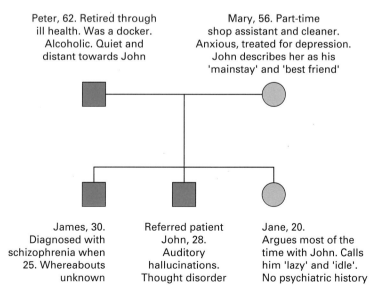

Peter, 62. Retired through ill health. Was a docker. Alcoholic. Quiet and distant towards John

Mary, 56. Part-time shop assistant and cleaner. Anxious, treated for depression. John describes her as his 'mainstay' and 'best friend'

James, 30. Diagnosed with schizophrenia when 25. Whereabouts unknown

Referred patient John, 28. Auditory hallucinations. Thought disorder

Jane, 20. Argues most of the time with John. Calls him 'lazy' and 'idle'. No psychiatric history

Fig. 1.1 John's family tree with family history notes.

Can they remember what it was like when they first went to school? Did they mix easily and find happiness with plenty of friends or were they lonely individuals, constantly being bullied? How did their parents get along? Were there numerous rows or was their home filled with mutual affection? If there were rows, did the child feel responsible for them in any way. Sometimes children feel that they cause marital breakdowns, especially if these occur at the 'age of magical thinking', i.e. when everything that happens in the outside world can be seen as a consequence of personal action. Examples of magical thinking include 'if I don't step on the lines in the pavement Mum and Dad will stay together'.

How did the person find the work at school — was it easy or was it very difficult for them? Were there any difficulties with reading delay or illiteracy? Were there any 'neurotic traits' such as prolonged bedwetting not due to organic causes, nailbiting, hair pulling, head-banging or encopresis?

When the time came to move from primary to secondary education, how was that transition? Was it a smooth and easy one or was it fraught with anxiety. Was any time taken off school for exaggerated illness (*school refusal*) or was their any truancy (with others or alone)? Did the person make new friends after the move? What were their favourite subjects at school? Any hobbies?

What qualifications or examinations did the person gain by the time they left school? This may give an indication of their intelligence level. What did they do after they left school? Put together a work history of where people worked, what they did and for how long. If they left a job, why did they leave? Was it because they were made redundant, got bored or found a better post? Were they fired because they were difficult personalities or because they were becoming mentally ill? In the early phases of illness people often underperform at work, especially in depression and schizophrenia. Because of their low self-esteem in depression, the depressed individual may think that their sacking is entirely justified and make no protest when in fact they are ill.

There are aspects of a person's life which they tend to keep to themselves unless they are prompted to talk about them. This may be because they are embarrassing aspects of their life or are aspects which will damage the way they are seen by others.

A person may not discuss their impotence because they feel embarrassed by this. Another person may choose not to disclose his conviction for fraud because it will colour what you think of them. One of the barriers to disclosure is if the patient feels that their doctor is easily embarrassed or does not wish to discuss sensitive aspects of their lives. Unfortunately, such sensitive aspects of people's lives are often the ones that cause them the most anxiety. Such patients suffer in silence. The doctor who shows a willingness to discuss such matters openly helps his or her patients disclose. Such aspects are often crucial to diagnosis and management and must not be ignored. At first you may feel embarrassed in such discussions but your discomfort will ease with experience. Two such areas that you will need to cover in the personal history are the patient's psychosexual history and their forensic history (or criminal record).

Psychosexual history

What relevance is a patient's sexual history? It is important to realise that sexuality is inherent in all people regardless of their age, physical well-being or mental condition and is a major factor in their lives. Psychosexual functioning seems to have some bearing on prognosis. Good function often correlates with a better prognosis. Sexual orientation is a problem for some people and this may provide a focus for psychotherapeutic interventions. Psychosexual function is also of value in making judgements about dangerousness in some sexual offenders. Psychiatrists are, therefore, interested in what kind of relationships the person builds up. *Schizoid* personalities tend to avoid contact with other people, especially sexual relationships, so their psychosexual history may be characterised by a complete absence or avoidance of sexuality. Their sexuality may, however, be expressed in isolation, by fantasy or masturbation. *Borderline* personalities sometimes have many intense but fleeting sexual relationships. The relationships may be affected by discord or violence. In depressive illness there is often a reduced sexual drive and this may cause difficulties with the partner. Similarly, mania may lead to a heightening of sexuality and a lack of judgement which may put patients at risk because they have unprotected sex with people they might not normally approach.

What is included in the psychosexual history? We wish to know generally about the patient's current and past loving relationships. Are they a source of general pleasure and satisfaction or are they characterised by rows or unhappiness? Specifically we need to know when the person began building relationships — at what age? What was their source of sexual education? What were their feelings about sex? How long did their first relationships last? Were they happy experiences or were there problems? How did they manage those problems? When was the first experience of sexual intercourse? Are the relationships heterosexual or homosexual? You need to know whether sex is pleasurable, merely satisfactory or if there are any specific sexual dysfunctions like impotence, vaginismus and premature ejaculation.

A history of childhood sexual abuse may affect an individual's capacity to enjoy subsequent sexual relationships and may also have relevance to abnormal personality development, alcoholism, eating disorders and depression. Some psychiatrists include a screening question for sexual abuse in all their initial interviews. It could take this form: 'These days more people seem able to talk about difficult things which have happened in their childhood. Some people are able to talk about how they were beaten as a child or how sometimes older people took advantage of them sexually. Has anything like that ever happened to you?' Other psychiatrists prefer to allow their patients to disclose at their own pace, although they create an atmosphere of trust and safety where the person can disclose what they wish when they wish. For some people disclosing past abuse is relatively easy, for others the disclosure and the fear of subsequent rejection by the doctor may make disclosure very threatening. Disclosures of ongoing abuse or violence, or where there is disclosure that a minor is at risk, may necessitate action to protect the individual or a third party.

Forensic history

The forensic history concerns the overlap between criminal offending behaviour and psychiatry and might be started by a question such as 'Have you ever been in trouble with the police?' You will need to record all charges and convictions, together with whether this ties in with periods of mental illness.

Social history

The social history needs to record information such as where the patient is living and who they are living with. How do they get on with these people? A hostile environment may predispose to relapse in certain psychiatric illnesses. Are there any financial problems? Finally, unless previously recorded, how much does the patient smoke and drink? Smoking is a long-term risk factor for depression. In relapse or in times of stress or anxiety, a smoker's tobacco consumption increases. Similarly, alcohol consumption may rise. People with alcohol problems are notoriously evasive about exactly how much they drink. You will need to press the point. Sometimes alcoholics are reluctant themselves to face up to how much they consume. How much do they drink a day? What time of day do they start drinking? When they wake do they have a tremor that goes away with the first drink of the morning? Have they ever had the DTs (delirium tremens), blackouts or fits? Withdrawal fits occur in up to 10% of alcoholics. Have they any memory problems? Failure to remember the events of the night before is sometimes referred to as a palimpsest, especially when the individual then begins to make up what they think happened the night before. These false memories are often likely things that might have happened. For example, an individual may tell you a long story about doing the washing that morning and hanging it out to dry in the back garden when in fact they have been on the ward all morning. The story is 'invented' to fill the gap in their memory which occurs because alcohol-induced brain damage has affected their ability to lay down new memories. The whole process of telling these false memories, which may appear valid to the individual, is known as confabulation. Ask also about street drugs use — what types, how often and how recently. Street drugs are linked to the development of short- and long-term psychoses. Besides street drugs you will need to take details of all currently prescribed drugs, with dosages and side-effects.

Premorbid personality

The penultimate history item is the premorbid personality. This is an idea of the patient's personality before the first signs of any mental illness. You can ask people to describe themselves as individuals. You may need to prompt them with adjectives such as shy, easy-going, nervous or extrovert. You might wish to probe for hobbies or interests, favourite books or films to build up a picture of the person opposite you.

Corroborative history

An individual's view of him or herself is necessarily subjective, so psychiatrists often ask for permission to speak to a relative or friend. This corroborative history might shed greater light on the patient's premorbid personality and how the illness has affected them. It will allow you to check details of alcohol and drug consumption. An important point to bear in mind is that in most cases you are taking information after gaining consent from the patient. You should not offer information to the relative or friend regarding other aspects of the history or diagnosis. There is a matter of confidentiality here. However, should the patient agree and want you to, such things may be discussed, but this probably should not arise during the history taking because your assessment and diagnosis is incomplete.

When the history is complete there are still other components of your assessment to be done, but this is a useful time to pause and take stock of things with the patient. A useful thing to do is to summarise the history back to the patient. This has two benefits: it enables the patient to correct any mistakes you have made and, therefore, clarify your view of things and it also allows the patient to feel understood by another person, sometimes for the first time in their lives. This exploration of how things have been can turn up new information and may offer some insight to the patient that they never had before. Some studies have found that patients do benefit from one-off interviews of this type.

The mental state examination

The mental state examination involves:

- eliciting psychological symptoms and signs
- recording these symptoms and signs in a systematic way.

This allows you to distinguish organic brain syndromes from other illnesses and to put evidence together to make a differential diagnosis.

The mental state examination is used in every assessment but, particularly when a patient is too ill to give a history, the mental state examination can be useful in making a diagnosis. The examination has a logical sequence to it so that the first item (appearance) can give evidence which affects the conduct of the rest of the examination, for instance if the patient appears to be unconscious or is very drowsy, assessment of mood or abstract thought is rendered unreliable or even worthless.

Components

The components of the mental state examination are:

- appearance
- behaviour
- manner
- speech
- mood
- thought
- cognition
- language
- insight.

Appearance

Briefly describe the patient's appearance, such as 'A thin 80-year-old man, smartly dressed in a three piece suit, carrying a leather bound Bible.' The description should not be a pejorative judgement of the person. You should be prepared to justify everything you ever write about a patient. Having said that, it is of great value to record exactly what you do see because this will influence your diagnosis and management. So that if you see a 'frail, elderly caucasian man, with grimy clothing and smelling of urine', then all these points may have some relevance — this appearance might suggest self-neglect, which can be a feature of general ill-health, depression or dementia. Other more bizarre features of appearance will need documentation, e.g. 'a 24-year-old man, wearing few clothes and with his head in a skull-cap of tin-foil, allegedly 'to keep out the cosmic rays', or 'a large 40-year-old lady, dressed only in a thin night-dress, standing in casualty, with her make-up over-liberally applied, and waving a bag of pig's trotters'. The former bizarre description accurately described a young man suffering from schizophrenia who had survived alone in a derelict flat for months eating raw meat and vegetables and the latter neatly fitted a lady with mania who had just been shopping in the local market. She had not felt the need to dress that morning and having grown tired of carefully applying her make-up, slapped it on.

Behaviour

The patient's behaviour may be altogether appropriate to the interview situation, he or she may sit quietly, answering each question carefully enough. Other patients may pace the room in an agitated way whilst the doctor tries to persuade them to stay in the room to answer more questions. Patients might leap out of their chair suddenly at the behest of unseen voices or they may be too preoccupied with visual hallucinations to concentrate on the doctor's questions. Some patients may appear unduly still, with their eyes unmoving and their limbs held tensely — these may be catatonic patients whose limbs if moved by the doctor may be put into unusual postures and have increased tone (*waxy flexibility* or *cereas flexibilitas*). The postures may then be held for minutes or hours (*preservation of posture*). Alternatively, the patient may be mute and still because they have psychomotor retardation, as in depression (this lacks the features of increased tone and abnormal posturing). It may be appropriate to include other movement disorders under behaviour and manner — psychotropic drugs sometimes cause restlessness (*akathisia*) or acute dystonic reactions (*torticollis, oculogyric crises* etc) or late-onset rhythmic involuntary lipsmacking, abnormal tongue movements, limb athetosis and truncal movements (*tardive dyskinesia*). Patients who mimic your every move are showing *echopraxia*.

Manner

Patients are usually cooperative in manner, but some may be suspicious, guarded or hostile to your questions. Record this. Also try and record how well you got on with the patient in terms of rapport.

Could you establish rapport with the patient? Could you both maintain eye contact or did the patient look down at the floor throughout the interview and answer questions reluctantly or not at all? Patients may also be over-friendly in manner (disinhibited as in mania) or over-hostile. Hostility may arise because patients are irritated with you or afraid of you — manic patients can be frustrated if you do not follow their fast thinking and paranoid patients may be suspicious of your motives and feel you are part of 'the plot'.

Speech

The speech of the patient may be totally spontaneous or may occur only when you ask questions. The answers to questions are usually relevant, but may be wildly off the point.

Sometimes all the patient's speech is spontaneous and irrelevant and any intervention by the doctor is unheeded. When answers to questions begin relevantly but drift from the point this may be termed circumstantial speech, e.g. in answer to a question about their mother's age at death: 'Well, she died young, not to say tragically, through an accident, I think there are too many accidents now. They're becoming more and more common. It's a violent world. Look at the gang wars about drugs . . . .' There is a conversational logic to this kind of speech, but it is difficult to focus in history-taking as the actual information that the patient's mother died at 45 is never given.

Alternatively, answers to questions may be given in the minutest detail: 'My normal working day? I get up at 7.36, and wash in the bathroom whilst listening to Radio 3. I shave with a razor. I like it better than an electric shaver. Then I get dressed in the clothes my wife has put out for me the night before. I like a newly ironed shirt every morning. Then I go downstairs and have two pieces of toast and a mug of freshly-brewed coffee . . .' This kind of speech is over-inclusive — there is just too much information.

Other speech types include tangential speech which veers markedly away from the topic under discussion and may be a feature of thought disordered speech. In mania speech may be pressured — the speech is rapid and crammed with ideas that tumble over one another to be expressed. In schizophrenia and some organic disorders there may be *perseverative* features such as the rhythmic repetition of the last words you said, known as *echolalia*, or the last syllable, *palilalia*.

Speech may be slowed down (as in psychomotor retardation). Speech disorders also include the results of brain damage (e.g. due to cerebrovascular ischaemia) which may produce dysarthrias, expressive and receptive dysphasias and word-finding difficulties.

Mood

The evidence derived from observations of appearance, behaviour, manner and speech can be used to form an idea of the patient's mood. The patient's affect during the interview may have been one of sadness or elation. The affect may have remained the same throughout the interview or it may have varied in response to your questions (it is normal for people to be sad when recalling past traumas and happy when sharing a joke). When people's affect changes suddenly and repeatedly without due cause this is known as *lability of affect*, which is sometimes a feature of organic brain damage. A patient's affect seems incongruous if it does not match the topic being discussed, e.g. laughter when discussing their mother's death. In patients with severe depression it may be difficult to see their affect because they are psychomotor retarded. The severely depressed person's face may lack emotional expression, sometimes called *flattened affect*. In schizophrenia the patient may complain that they never feel highs or lows in their mood (*blunted affect*).

Using what you have found during the preceding assessment you can now build up an 'objective' view of the patient's mood, with the evidence to back this up. Ask the patient for their 'subjective' view of their mood and record this. A suitable question might be: 'Can you tell me how you've been feeling, in your mood or in your spirits, over the past few days or weeks?' You might like to give prompts such as 'High or low? Sad or happy?' If they give a reply of sad or happy try and gauge whether this has been excessive: e.g. 'How sad?' or 'The saddest you've ever been?' And in all patients probe for any suicidal ideation, 'Have you ever felt life was not worth living? Have you felt like this recently?' And if the answers are 'yes', then ask, 'Have you thought of doing anything about that?

Have you got any plans to harm yourself? How would you kill yourself? When would you do it? What might stop you doing that?'

Also record again any biological features of mood disturbance: sleep abnormalities (initial insomnia, waking and early morning wakening), poor appetite, weight loss (exactly how much?), diurnal mood variation, altered sexual drive and constipation.

Thought

In the section on thought we are concerned with two main headings: *form* and *content*. The form of thought may be reflected by speech. Thus if speech is thought disordered it may be reasonable to assume that thought (which occurs before speech) is similarly disordered. Thoughts may also be pressured, which may lead to pressure of speech, they may be dominated by intrusive thoughts (as in obsessive compulsive disorder), they may exhibit flights of ideas (as in mania) or sudden unpleasant gaps (as in thought blocking in schizophrenia). In the content of thought you might ask for the main thoughts that dominate a person's recent thinking life: 'What kind of things do you think about most?', 'What kind of things do you worry about nowadays?' Record any worries, preoccupations, intrusive thoughts, over-valued ideas or delusions. Under thought content you may also record any abnormal experiences such as hallucinatory experiences or thought interference (withdrawal, insertion or broadcasting).

Cognition

Cognitive testing seeks to elicit signs that may point to an organic psychiatric disease. For instance, in a hallucinated patient if consciousness is diminished or 'clouded' then this may mean that the hallucinations are the product of a delirious state (acute organic brain syndrome) perhaps due to infection or hypoxia. If there are memory problems on cognitive testing then it may be that there is a dementing process at work.

A basic scheme for cognitive testing might be:

- **Orientation**. Normally in daytime people are aware of the time, the place they are in and the people they are with. In organic brain syndrome this orientation to time, place and person is gradually lost. It is possible to be disorientated just in time or disorientated in all three. Ask for the current date (day, date, month, year) and the time of day. Ask for the place — 'Where are we now?' — find out if the patient knows which ward, hospital or clinic they are in. Finally do they know who you are or do they imagine you to be a priest or a social worker (assuming that you have introduced yourself properly at some time during the interview)?

- **Attention and concentration.** An inability to focus attention may be seen in agitated depression, anxiety, mania or organic syndromes. Tests which can be used include: 'Please say the months of the year for me in reverse order, that is working backwards from December through to January . . .' or 'Please say the days of the week in reverse order, staring with Sunday and working back to Monday', or 'please take 7 away from 100, now carry on taking 7 away from that, and again . . . . (known as 'serial 7s') or 'please take 3 away from 21 and keep on taking 3 away until there is nothing left'. Other tests may include digit spans — seeing how many numbers an individual can repeat back to you in sequence or reverse sequence, e.g. 364 . . . . . 463, 7924 . . . . . 4297. These tests help you assess attention, but do involve other skills too, so that if these other skills are lost then it may appear that attention is poor when it is not. If someone is poor at maths or has a specific brain defect which causes dyscalculia (a parietal lobe deficit) then serial 7s or serial 3s will not produce useful results.

- **Memory.** Some people define short-term memory as everything remembered up to 3 minutes ago and everything retained beyond 3 minutes or so as medium- or long-term memory. Definitions of short- and long-term memory are contentious and you will observe that different psychiatrists and psychologists have different ideas about this. In a basic cognitive screening we are interested in fairly crude tests of memory function — short-term testing may involve asking someone to remember a new name and address. 'I would like you to listen to and remember a new name and address I am going to say to you. I will repeat it until you are happy you have got it in mind.' The name and address may have, say, seven compo-

nents. See initially how many times you have to repeat the name and address before the individual can repeat it back word perfect (i.e. how many times does it take before they register the address). Then ask them to recall the address at fixed intervals, for example 30 seconds, 1 minute, 3 minutes and 5 minutes and then record how many components they can give back to you:

	30 seconds	1 minute	3 minutes	5 minutes
Number of address components	7/7	6/7	4/7	2/7

This gives you an 'objective' measure of memory function which you can use for later comparison. Other short-term tests might include giving a list of five different objects and asking the individual to repeat these back to you at certain times. You will also need to get an idea of long-term memory function — can the individual recall important personal dates (e.g. birthdays and anniversaries) — although this is only useful if you have an objective source to check these with. Otherwise, use the dates of important historical events such as the dates of the Second World War, the death of Churchill, the date of the first moon landing, etc. You can sometimes ask for the names of five flowers, five animals or five capital cities. Short-term memory function deteriorates first in dementia syndromes, but all these memory tests may be affected in severe dementia or by mental retardation.

Language

You may ask patients with suspected dementia to name readily available items, such as a pen, a watch or a chair. An impairment of naming and word-finding is often an early sign of dementia. Other language skills can be tested by asking the patient to follow simple instructions, e.g. 'use your right hand to touch the tip of your nose'. Ask the patient to register and repeat simple and more complicated sentences, e.g. 'The one thing that a nation needs is a large and secure supply of wood.' Finally, make an assessment of reading a short paragraph and writing a short sentence.

Cerebral lobe function

If the cognitive screening has been normal up to now then it is probably not of use to probe further into cerebral lobe function, but if a dementia syndrome seems likely then some simple tests may be useful in determining whether there is frontal or parietal lobe damage.

A simple test for frontal lobe damage seeks to assess whether there are any perseverative tendencies. The patient is asked to copy a rhythmically changing line pattern. With some frontal lobe lesions the patient may perseverate as in Figure 1.2. Perseveration of actions such as in drawing or in speech is often linked with frontal lesions.

Other tests for frontal lobe function include *verbal fluency*, where the subject is asked to give as many words as possible in a minute beginning with the letter 'F', 'A' and then 'S'. For the 'FAS' verbal fluency test normal subjects score > 30 in total; a score of 20–30 denotes mild frontal dysfunction and a score < 20 suggest large, frontal lesions or a dementing illness.

Interpreting proverbs is an example of *abstracting ability* and with frontal lobe lesions patients may interpret proverbs in a 'concrete' way. For example in interpreting 'A rolling stone gathers no moss' a frontal lobe patient may say that 'The stone gathers no moss because it is moving too fast.'

Paper tests for parietal lobe damage may seek to assess whether there is a constructional apraxia. When asked to copy a line drawing of a house or a

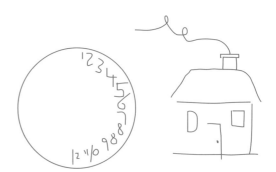

Fig. 1.3 The results of asking a patient with unilateral spatial neglect to draw a clock face and copy a simple drawing of a house.

clock, the copy may be 'exploded', or there may be sensory inattention to one side of the diagram (Fig. 1.3).

Abstract thought

In schizophrenia, mental retardation and frontal lesions the capacity for abstract thinking may be reduced, so that concrete thinking is prevalent. Tests for abstract thought may therefore include asking for the meaning of proverbs or for asking for similarities between things such as a banana and an apple (correct answer: 'both fruits' or 'both living things') or a car and a lorry, or for differences between things like a lake and a river or a child and a dwarf. Such tests may also provoke thought disorder in some predisposed individuals.

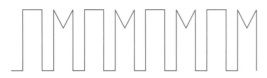

Rhythmically changing line pattern

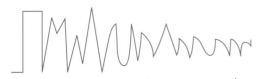

Copy of line pattern showing perseveration

Fig. 1.2 In copying a regularly changing line pattern the patient with perseveration fails to change the pattern and continues in zig-zag fashion.

Insight

Finally, the interviewer assesses the patient's 'insight' into their illness — does the patient think they have any problems and if so are they due to ill-health, do they think that the illness is treatable by doctors, and is it treatable by drugs? Psychotic illnesses often rob patients of insight so that they feel their voices are normal, or supernaturally derived, or attributable to some alien authority rather than being due to a treatable illness. If they make this assumption about their psychotic experiences and delusions then it would be illogical for the patient to think that doctors can help. Lack of insight may reduce or destroy the patient's compliance with treatment and, without outside intervention, condemn the mentally ill to permanent ill-health.

Insight is, therefore, about how the patient sees their predicament and is a complex construct.

Physical examination and investigations

Psychiatrists are first and foremost doctors, trained in diagnosis and keen to exclude any treatable physical illness which may present with psychological symptoms. A routine physical examination of cardiovascular, respiratory, abdominal and nervous systems is, therefore, essential in all patients. Organic causes of psychiatric illness which may be picked up in this way might include: focal CNS lesions, subdural haematomas, SLE, hyperthyroidism, hypothyroidism, diabetes mellitus, Addison's, Cushing's, hypertension, renal and liver failure, phaeocromocytomas, tuberose sclerosis, syphilis, bronchial and gastric carcinomas, stigmata of alcoholic liver disease, features of mental retardation syndromes, e.g. Down or Fragile-X, and numerous others.

Similarly, investigations may usefully include a full blood count (various anaemias may present with dementia-like pictures, raised mean cell volume in alcoholism), liver enzyme tests (raised in alcoholism), thyroid function tests, serum B_{12} and folate, urea and electrolytes, syphilis screening tests, drug screening tests (street drugs may induce psychotic reactions), chest X-ray, skull X-rays, electroencephalogram (to detect focal lesions and epileptic phenomena), computed tomography/ magnetic resonance scans, and more specialist tests, e.g. cortisol levels, dexamethasone suppression tests, homovanillic acid urine tests, serum copper tests (for Wilson's disease).

Other investigations include social, occupational and psychological investigations. Social investigations (if consented to) may include discussions with family and friends, requests to schools for information on progress and abilities, home visits and the like. Occupational therapists may assist with rehabilitation as will functional assessments (how well people can manage their home life and plan their daily activities). Psychologists can sometime help with specific neuropsychological tests of brain function and personality and IQ testing.

Putting the information together

At the end of the assessment process the doctor pulls together the major findings from the history, mental state, physical examination and investigations into a summary. Sometimes the summary is built into a 'formulation' which also includes a differential diagnosis and a tentative management plan and prognosis. The differential diagnosis should include the most likely diagnoses, headed by the most likely of all, together with evidence extracted from the assessment interview to support or refute each diagnosis. Using the differential diagnosis you can then, and only then, reasonably construct a management plan and prognosis which can be appended to the formulation.

In making your differential diagnosis you may wish to consider five 'levels of illness' in a sort of diagnostic sieve. The first level to consider is organic; specifically ask yourself if there is any organic illness that might present with such features. This must be included in your differential diagnosis and steps taken to exclude treatable organic illness. It makes little sense to embark on psychological methods of treatment without treating underlying organic causes. The second level is 'affective illness', by which we mean illnesses with affective features (such as mania or depression) which are not caused by gross organic disorder (such as delirium or intracerebral tumours or infarctions). The third level would be schizophrenic illness. The fourth level is 'neurotic' illness which encompasses minor disturbances of mood, anxiety disorders, phobias and eating disorders. Such illnesses may be very disabling, but they lack psychotic features. Finally, the fifth area to consider involves the personality. People's personalities differ to a greater or lesser extent. When those differences are marked, persistent and damaging to the individual or society they are termed *personality disorders*. Some personality disorders may mimic other psychiatric illness but it is worth bearing in mind that just as all personality types can become physically ill, so all personality types can suffer from psychiatric illness. It would be unethical to deny treatment to someone purely on the basis that they had a personality disorder.

Classification

Classifying disease helps doctors to recognise clinically similar illnesses in people and enables research, particularly in terms of what causes those illnesses and what cures them. In psychiatry large groups have met to define illness categories and currently there are two broad classification systems in use. The European and world-wide system is the International Classification of Diseases, 10th version, (ICD-10) and the American system is the Diagnostic and Statistical Manual, 4th version (DSM-IV). There is substantial overlap between them. When you make a diagnosis according to the criteria for each disease in these classifications then other clinicians will be able to know what you mean when you diagnose schizophrenia.

A useful thumbnail classification to have in mind when interviewing a patent is the one in the psychiatric 'sieve' above: organic, affective, schizophrenic, neurotic and personality disorders. However, when making a formal presentation the following classification may be of use, especially if read in conjunction with the relevant chapters. Although one diagnosis may take precedence, remember that several diagnoses may be present, e.g. depression in a patient with residual schizophrenia or depression in a person with borderline personality disorder.

In the following section the main headings of ICD-10 are summarised. At this stage you may not be familiar with all the terms mentioned, but reference to the following chapters will help you.

ICD-10

F00–F09

- **Organic mental disorders**
  Examples include:
  — Dementia in Alzheimer's disease — may be early or late onset. Vascular dementia (includes acute, multi-infarct, and subcortical types)
  — Dementia in the following: Pick's disease; Creutzfeldt-Jakob disease; Huntington's chorea; Parkinson's disease; and HIV infection/AIDS.
  — Delirium (an acute organic brain syndrome with disorientation and clouding of consciousness)
  — Organic hallucinosis, e.g. caused by temporal lobe epilepsy, organic mood disorders, e.g. in Cushing's syndrome, organic anxiety disorders, e.g. in phaeochromocytoma.
- **Organic personality disorder**, e.g. frontal lobe tumours which may disorganise personality, postencephalitic syndromes and postconcussional syndromes.

F10–F19 Mental and behavioural disorders due to psychoactive substance abuse

- This covers alcohol, opioids, cannabinoids, sedatives, hypnotics, cocaine, caffeine, amphetamines, other hallucinogens, tobacco, solvents and other drugs.
- May include harmful use, dependence, withdrawal states, psychotic disorders, e.g. delirium tremens and LSD experiences, amnesic syndromes, e.g. Wernicke-Korsakoff syndrome, and residual effects, e.g. LSD flashbacks.

F20–29 Schizophrenia, schizotypal and delusional disorders

- Schizophrenia (this may take the form of paranoid, hebephrenic, catatonic, undifferentiated, or residual types)
- Schizotypal disorder (this lacks the full psychotic features of schizophrenia — it is more of an extreme of personality featuring unusual or eccentric ideation, for instance, magical thinking)
- Persistent delusional disorders, e.g. monodelusional psychoses where the individual wrongly believes they are, say, infested by some insect, but no other psychotic features
- Schizoaffective disorder — a rare category where the illness has marked features of both affective illness and schizophrenia.

F30–F39 Mood (affective) disorders

- Manic episode (which would include hypomania — a lesser form of mania and probably more common; mania without psychotic features; and mania with psychotic features)
- Bipolar affective disorder (this diagnosis requires evidence of both hypomanic or manic and depressive episodes at some stage in a person's life)
- Depressive episodes (which can be categorised as mild, moderate and severe without depressive symptoms and severe with psychotic symptoms)
- Recurrent mood disorders

- Persistent mood disorders (cyclothymia — a varying series of low and high moods, dysthymia — a chronic, low mood not severe enough to fulfil the criteria for a depressive illness).

F40–F48 Neurotic, stress-related and somatoform disorders

- Phobic anxiety disorders (such as agoraphobia, social phobias, specific phobias)
- Anxiety disorders (such as panic disorder, generalised anxiety disorder)
- Obsessive-compulsive disorder (involving obsessional thoughts or ruminations, compulsive acts and obsessional rituals)
- Reactions to severe stress and adjustment disorders
- Dissociative (conversion) disorders — where some internal conflict or anxiety is converted into other symptoms like classical Freudian hysterical paralysis. Examples of dissociative disorders include dissociative amnesias, dissociative fugues, trance and possession states, dissociative convulsions and dissociative anaesthesia
- Somatoform disorders — somatising anxiety into any physical symptom
- Depersonalisation-derealisation syndrome.

F50–F59 Behavioural syndromes associated with physiological disturbances and physical factors

- Eating disorders (anorexia nervosa, bulimia nervosa and others)
- Non-organic sleep disorders (where organic causes have been excluded — insomnia, hypersomnia, somnambulism, night terrors, nightmares)
- Sexual dysfunction (not caused by organic disorder or disease) (includes — loss of sexual desire, sexual aversion, failure of genital response, orgasmic dysfunction, premature ejaculation, non-organic vaginismus, non-organic dyspareunia, excessive sexual drive and others)
- Mental and behavioural disorders of the puerperium
- Abuse of non-dependence producing substances (like laxatives, analgesics, antacids, vitamins etc.).

F60–69 Disorders of adult personality and behaviour

- Personality disorders (including paranoid, schizoid, dissocial, borderline, histrionic, anankastic, avoidant, dependent and other types)

- Enduring personality change after catastrophic experience or psychiatric illness
- Pathological gambling, firesetting, stealing, hair-pulling.
- Transsexualism, dual-role transvestism
- Sexual preference disorders — fetishism, exhibitionism, voyeurism, paedophilia, sadomasochism etc.
- Factitious disorder (intentional feigning of symptoms or disabilities), sometimes also called Munchausen's syndrome.

F70–F79 Mental retardation

- Mild, moderate, severe and profound.

F80–F89 Disorders of psychological development

- Developmental disorders of speech, receptive and expressive language disorders, specific arithmetical disorders
- Childhood autism, Rett's syndrome, Asperger's syndrome.

F90–F98 Behavioural and emotional disorders with onset usually occurring in childhood and adolescence

- Hyperkinetic disorders, conduct disorders, emotional disorders, tic disorders, non-organic enuresis, non-organic encopresis, pica, stereotyped movement disorders, stuttering.

F99 Unspecified mental disorder

LEARNING POINTS

Psychiatric assessment

- A psychiatric assessment has four main components: history, mental state examination, physical examination and investigations (physical, psychological and social).
- The history is divided into presenting complaint, the history of presenting complaint, past psychiatric history, family history, personal history, psychosexual history, forensic history, social history, premorbid personality, corroborative history and summary.
- The mental state examination describes appearance, behaviour and manner, speech, mood (including suicidal feelings), thought (form and content), cognition and insight.

Self-assessment

MCQs

1 Clinical features of depression typically include:
  a psychomotor retardation
  b diurnal mood variation
  c early morning wakening
  d overactivity
  e constipation

2 Routine first line psychiatric investigations include:
  a full blood count
  b magnetic resonance imaging
  c serum copper
  d thyroid function tests
  e liver function tests

3 Types of personality disorder include:
  a schizoid
  b residual
  c blunted
  d borderline
  e hebephrenic

4 In the following mental state abnormalities:
  a echolalia is the copying of posture
  b tangentiality may occur in thought disorder
  c overvalued ideas are incorrect, unreasonable and bizarre ideas held with absolute conviction
  d word finding difficulties are a feature of early dementia
  e hallucinatory voices talking to the patient are third person auditory hallucinations

Short answer questions

1 What are the differences between a hallucination and an illusion?
2 What are the main features of a delusion? What different kinds of delusion are there?
3 What cognitive tests help to assess someone's attention and concentration? How do you perform these tests?

MCQ answers

1 a = T,　b = T,　c = T,　d = F,　e = T
2 a = T,　b = F,　c = F,　d = T,　e = T
3 a = T,　b = F,　c = F,　d = T,　e = F
4 a = F,　b = T,　c = F,　d = T,　e = F

Further reading and references

FISH F 1977 In: Hamilton M (ed) Clinical Psychopathology. Wright, Bristol

GREEN B H 1994 Creating Rapport. In: Green (ed) Psychiatry in General Practice. Kluwer Academic Publishers, London

JASPERS K 1959 General Psychopathology. Manchester University Press, Manchester

SHEA S C 1988 Psychiatric Interviewing. Saunders, Philadelphia

SIMS A 1988 Symptoms in the Mind. Bailliere Tindall, London

WORLD HEALTH ORGANIZATION 1992 The ICD-10 Classification of Mental and Behavioural Disorders. WHO, Geneva

2

Organic psychiatry

The body's homeostatic mechanisms strive to create a supportive environment for the brain. These mechanisms regulate blood pressure so that the brain is adequately perfused with blood rich in glucose and oxygen. If untoward problems occur, such as metabolic disease, infection or starvation, other body systems will be denied in order to preserve the life of the brain. However, if these problems are sufficiently severe the homeostatic mechanisms will be overwhelmed and brain function will suffer.

The presentation of this organic illness may well be through psychological symptoms, but management must aim to identify the cause of the cerebral disorder and to treat this where possible. Failure to treat the underlying cause will increase the risk of death.

Contents

A review of brain function

The brain consists of a cluster of structures which have evolved over time. Some structures such as the *brainstem* are relatively ancient in evolutionary terms and perform necessary but rudimentary functions such as coordinating respiratory rhythm and fulfilling basic aims of life such as consciousness. Higher, later structures such as the *white matter* allow the functions of association and learning. Relatively new structures such as the *cortex* allow the integration of sensations, ideas and movements

and form the core of sentient cognition. *Forebrain* structures in the frontal lobes of the brain allow finer functions still such as judgement, insight and detailed planning.

Psychological symptoms may be produced by lesions which affect any or all brain components.

Figure 2.1 shows how various functions correspond to different areas of the cerebral cortex. Left and right hemispheres also appear to have different roles. In over 90% of people the left hemisphere houses the language centres and controls handedness. Certain functions are shared out between the hemispheres via the integrative ability of the corpus

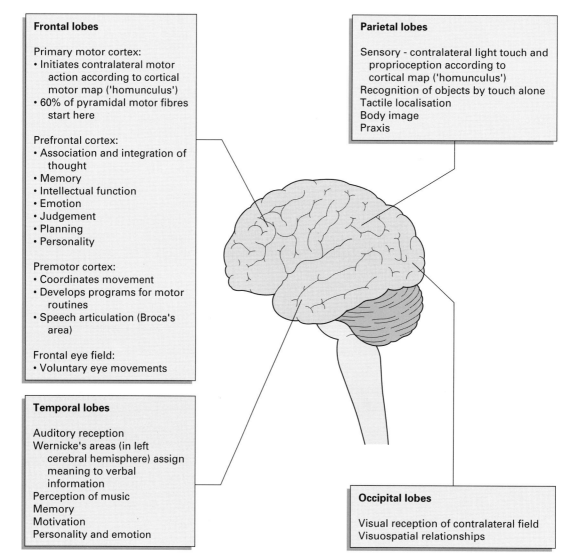

Frontal lobes

Primary motor cortex:
• Initiates contralateral motor action according to cortical motor map ('homunculus')
• 60% of pyramidal motor fibres start here

Prefrontal cortex:
• Association and integration of thought
• Memory
• Intellectual function
• Emotion
• Judgement
• Planning
• Personality

Premotor cortex:
• Coordinates movement
• Develops programs for motor routines
• Speech articulation (Broca's area)

Frontal eye field:
• Voluntary eye movements

Temporal lobes

Auditory reception
Wernicke's areas (in left cerebral hemisphere) assign meaning to verbal information
Perception of music
Memory
Motivation
Personality and emotion

Parietal lobes

Sensory - contralateral light touch and proprioception according to cortical map ('homunculus')
Recognition of objects by touch alone
Tactile localisation
Body image
Praxis

Occipital lobes

Visual reception of contralateral field
Visuospatial relationships

Fig. 2.1 Normal functions related to different cerebral lobes.

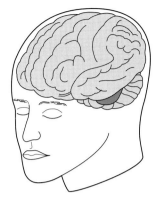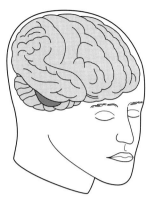

Left
Language
Handedness
Movement of right
  side of body
Sensory information from
  right side of body
Visual reception of right
  visual field
Verbal memory
Bilateral auditory
  reception
Processing of verbal
  sound
Visuo-verbal processing

Right
Movement of left side of
  body
Sensory information
  from left side of body
Visual reception of left
  visual field
Non-verbal memory, e.g.
  pictures, patterns
Bilateral auditory
  reception
Processing of music,
  noise
Visuo-spatial
  processing
Emotional processing

Fig. 2.2 Functions of the right and left sides of the brain.

callosum. Figure 2.2 indicates the differing functions of left and right hemispheres.

General conditions, such as hypoglycaemia or hypoxia, alter the function of all parts of the brain. Effects on the frontal lobe may produce disinhibition and impaired judgement and effects on the temporal lobe may lead to hallucinatory experiences. Effects on general neural activity may result in diminished consciousness so that, for example, the hypoxic elderly patient may appear drowsy but also experience frightening hallucinations and be unable to distinguish what is real and what is unreal around her. Specific space-occupying lesions such as tumours or abscesses may produce symptoms only in the brain areas they impinge upon. Early symptoms of a frontal lobe tumour may involve fairly subtle changes in personality such as a slight coarseness of manner in a previously urbane and polite character. Figure 2.3 shows how lesions in various cerebral lobes may present. Depending on the size and type of the lesion

none, some or all of these symptoms and signs may occur.

Appreciation of how organic disease can affect brain function helps provide a link between the symptoms of a psychiatric disease such as senile dementia and the neuropathology that underlies it.

Causes of cerebral disorder

In general we might think of causes in terms of *vulnerability* and *stress*. If the stress is sufficient any brain will cease to function correctly, so a young adult who acquires malaria may suffer from *delirium* (an acute organic brain syndrome). Some brains are more vulnerable and may succumb to lesser stresses. A general anaesthetic may prove harmless to a young adult brain but, to the more vulnerable brain of an otherwise fit 90 year old, the stress of general anaesthesia may result in temporary disorientation postoperatively.

Accumulated brain cell death, diminished cardio-

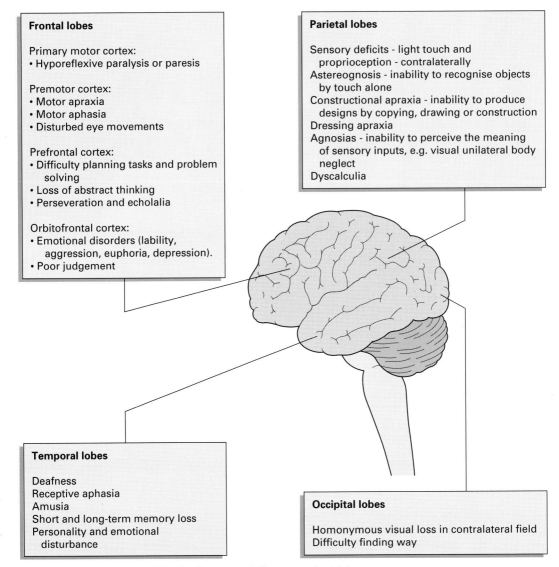

Frontal lobes

Primary motor cortex:
• Hyporeflexive paralysis or paresis

Premotor cortex:
• Motor apraxia
• Motor aphasia
• Disturbed eye movements

Prefrontal cortex:
• Difficulty planning tasks and problem
   solving
• Loss of abstract thinking
• Perseveration and echolalia

Orbitofrontal cortex:
• Emotional disorders (lability,
   aggression, euphoria, depression).
• Poor judgement

Parietal lobes

Sensory deficits - light touch and
   proprioception - contralaterally
Astereognosis - inability to recognise objects
   by touch alone
Constructional apraxia - inability to produce
   designs by copying, drawing or construction
Dressing apraxia
Agnosias - inability to perceive the meaning
   of sensory inputs, e.g. visual unilateral body
   neglect
Dyscalculia

Temporal lobes

Deafness
Receptive aphasia
Amusia
Short and long-term memory loss
Personality and emotional
   disturbance

Occipital lobes

Homonymous visual loss in contralateral field
Difficulty finding way

Fig. 2.3 Symptoms and signs related to lesions in different cerebral lobes.

vascular performance and other factors such as pigment deposition, neurofibrillary tangles and senile plaque formation all contribute to an increased vulnerability for older brains. Chronic degenerative disease in older brains may lead to a chronic brain syndrome called *dementia*.

Stresses that can produce brain dysfunction are listed in Table 2.1.

Delirium and dementia

Delirium is an *acute* brain syndrome. Key features that help distinguish it from traditional psychiatric illnesses are that it involves disorientation in time, place or person and a reduced level of consciousness. The level of consciousness may fluctuate with the underlying physical illness. The patient may also misinterpret the environment: illusions are common and hallucinations may occur. Delirium often occurs suddenly and is more likely to occur in vulnerable brains. *Delirium tremens* (or DTs) is an acute organic brain syndrome which may occur 3–5 days after alcohol dependent people stop drinking, e.g. shortly after they have been admitted to hos-

Table 2.1 Stresses that can induce cerebral disorder

Cerebro-vascular insufficiency	Heart failure, e.g. rhythm disturbance or myocardial infarction Pneumonitis Obstructive airways disease
Infections	Direct CNS infections Viral e.g. Epstein-Barr, Varicella zoster, HIV Bacterial e.g. Tuberculosis Fungal e.g. Cryptosporidium Protozoal e.g. Entamoeba histolyticum Toxins produced by distant infection
Tumour	Primaries (such as meningiomas) Secondaries (e.g. breast and lung)
Metabolic	Hypoglycaemia Hyperglycaemia Electrolyte disturbance, e.g. hyponatraemia
Endocrine	Hypothyroidism Hyperthyroidism Addisonian crisis Cushing's syndrome Parathyroid instability
Epilepsy	Auras and post-ictal phenomena Temporal lobe epilepsy Epileptogenic foci
Iatrogenic	Digoxin Histamine blockers Diuretics Beta-blockers and many other drugs in therapeutic and excess dosage

pital. The DTs are characterised by fearful illusions or, occasionally, hallucinations, classically of small creatures or figures (so-called Lilliputian hallucinations after the little people of Lilliput in *Gulliver's Travels*). The DTs is associated with a considerable mortality of 10% and requires careful medical management.

Dementia is a *chronic* brain syndrome. Disorientation is a likely feature but is not essential. The key feature is a history of progressive global cognitive decline over weeks and months. Inability to learn new material (loss of short-term memory) is seen as a hallmark of dementia. Dementia may be caused by a variety of cerebral and systemic diseases.

Dementia is often caused by Alzheimer's disease. Dementia caused by a succession of strokes is called multi-infarct dementia.

In younger patients dementia may be produced by inherited conditions such as Huntington's chorea and Wilson's disease, infections such as HIV or the consequences of alcoholism.

LEARNING POINTS

Cerebral disorder and organic psychiatry

- Psychological symptoms may be caused by general stresses such as metabolic disease or specific stresses such as cerebral tumours.
- Some brains are made more vulnerable to stresses through neuronal loss or disease. Stress may therefore produce cerebral dysfunction in one person and not in another.
- Specific stresses produce symptoms according to the site of the lesion. There are some syndromes associated with certain cerebral lobes.
- Frontal lobe syndrome includes changes in personality, poor judgement, social disinhibition, lability of mood, poor planning and loss of abstract thought. It may mimic psychiatric illnesses like hypomania.
- Delirium (acute organic brain syndrome) is an acute brain dysfunction which involves impaired consciousness, disorientation and misperception of the world around one. Dementia (chronic organic brain syndrome) is a chronic global deterioration of cognitive abilities occurring in clear consciousness.
- Features which should alert the doctor to organic brain syndromes are disorientation, fluctuating or impaired consciousness, illusions, visual hallucinations and intermittent periods of lucidity.
- Treatment of organic brain disease is by establishing the cause rather than sedation. Delirium may herald the patient's imminent death.

Case histories

CASE HISTORY 1

The family doctor was summoned by Mrs Jones'

daughter at 2 a.m. The daughter met the doctor at the front door of her mother's house. She told the doctor how her 78-year-old mother had been unwell for the past week with flu. In the last 2 days her mother had stayed in the bedroom all day, but had become agitated as night drew on. Mrs Jones had phoned her daughter (who lived two roads away) at 2 a.m. the previous day complaining that a burglar was trying to get into bed with her. When her daughter and son-in-law hurried round to help they found that there was no sign of a burglar and no sign of a break-in. Mr Jones had appeared confused and called her daughter by her own sister's name. She had been very restless through the night, but as dawn came she appeared less disturbed.

The daughter had called the doctor in the early hours because her mother had phoned her at midnight saying that a black mass was being held in the house opposite. When her daughter arrived she saw that Mrs Jones was talking about a man working on his car in the garage across the road. Mrs Jones described the lights in the garage as 'candles held by witches', who she said were 'chanting swear words'. The daughter had to wrestle her frightened mother back into bed. The daughter was very worried because her mother had never been like this before and had never seen a psychiatrist in her life.

What are the key features that point towards an acute organic brain syndrome?

The history gives a probable stress factor — a recent infection — possibly a bacterial infection superimposed on influenza. Mrs Jones' age makes her brain more vulnerable and as her consciousness fluctuates she becomes disorientated and misperceives reality. She perceives the man working on his car across the road as a 'black mass'. This is an example of a misinterpretation.

What are the main points to consider in this patient's management?

If there is an underlying bacterial infection this will need treatment, but the doctor will need to exclude other physical illnesses as well. A physical examination and investigations such as a chest X-ray, full

blood count, urea and electrolytes, random serum glucose and ECG would all be useful. Admission to hospital would be appropriate.

CASE HISTORY 2

Mr Dowling, 65, was brought to the accident and emergency department early one Saturday morning. He had been depressed for several weeks and had been talking about the pointlessness of life. Late on Friday night he had begun confusing his wife with his sister and talking about events that had happened 20 years ago as if they were only yesterday. He had suddenly become very frightened and said that a man with very long legs was standing in the living room beckoning him. His wife had been alarmed because she was in the room at the time and couldn't see what her husband was staring at. The psychiatry registrar was called to see the patient and took a careful history. The most important point in the history as far as the registrar was concerned was the fact that Mr Dowling had just been put on a tricyclic antidepressant by his family doctor.

Is this severe depression or delirium? What features are not typical of a severe depression and more typical of delirium?

Although it is possible for people with depression to become psychotic and have hallucinatory experiences, it is important to distinguish a psychotic depression from a delirium overlying a longstanding depression. The important points are the sudden change in the illness — Mr Dowling suddenly begins to be disorientated (mistaking his wife for his sister) and suddenly begins to have visual hallucinations. Visual hallucinations are strongly suggestive of an organic state. Taken together with the prescription of a drug that day would suggest a possible link between the two.

What is the likely cause of the delirium?

Tricyclic antidepressants affect various neurotransmitter systems including noradrenergic, serotonergic, histaminergic and cholinergic systems. The effects on cholinergic systems can induce hallucinatory experiences. It is obviously important to distinguish the delirium from a depressive psychosis because in the former you would discontinue the antidepressants whereas in the latter you would continue them (and probably perpetuate the delirium).

CASE HISTORY 3

Emma, 19, came to see her family doctor because occasionally she had episodes where she felt very unwell. The episodes started with rumblings in her stomach and palpitations. She often felt very frightened because these would go on for a few minutes, then she would see a blinding flash of light. Once she had heard someone talking to her for a few seconds. The voice had said, in a very strong tone, 'Fear is the key!'. She had been so frightened that she couldn't tell anyone and had gone on regardless, hoping that it wouldn't happen again.

Unfortunately the voice came back 2 weeks later after she had been out all night at a party. This time it said, 'It is nobler to suffer silently.' After these extraordinary experiences Emma felt very tired and often found that she could not concentrate on her school work. Her family were worried because her university exams were coming up and they said that sometimes she seemed so 'vague'. Emma was very worried she was 'going mad'.

What pointers are there to an organic illness?

There is a fluctuating history. Most of the time Emma is well with the illness occurring in discrete episodes. The episodes begin with autonomic symptoms like palpitations and gastrointestinal rumbling, focus in brief visual or auditory hallucinations and are followed by a variable period of lassitude and reduced consciousness. This episodic history is not like the mainly continuous symptoms in schizophrenia but is more suggestive of epilepsy. Temporal lobe epilepsy (TLE) often produces symptoms suggestive of schizophrenia but in this episodic way. Like other epilepsies TLE is more common when people are psychologically stressed (Emma is coming up for her exams) and when they

are physiologically stressed, e.g. when Emma is tired or maybe even hypoglycaemic after the party and alcohol.

There is also a possibility that Emma may have been experimenting with drugs, and drug-induced experiences would have to be excluded by a careful history and a relevant drug screen.

Emma's management would include a physical examination, routine blood investigations and an electroencephalogram (EEG) to try and confirm the diagnosis of TLE. Sometimes TLE is a difficult diagnosis to confirm and a referral to a neurologist would be appropriate. If the diagnosis of TLE appears to be correct, advice about lifestyle and the prescription of an antiepileptic drug like carbamazepine may be effective.

LEARNING POINTS

Case histories

- The management of organic brain syndromes relies upon a full history, physical examination and a range of investigations. Several causes may be present simultaneously.
- A careful drug history may reveal items that depress consciousness or act on specific neurotransmitters that may provoke cerebral disorder, e.g. dopamine agonists or anticholinergics.
- Temporal lobe epilepsy may induce various psychotic symptoms including hallucinations. The course of the history is usually episodic rather than continuous. An EEG may help in the diagnosis. Antiepileptic drugs are the treatment of choice.

Self-assessment

Cases

Read through the three cases that follow. As you read them ask yourself which illnesses might fit with these clinical presentations? Ask yourself how you would investigate these cases.

The answer section gives the actual diagnoses.

1 Mrs Alberta, 60, had been finding it difficult to concentrate on books and newspapers for a few weeks. Her thinking somehow felt different to her — less clear — and she was becoming much more forgetful.

Her daughter had noticed how tired and sluggish Mrs Alberta had become. From being an active pensioner who had helped in the local church coffee shop every day, Mrs Alberta had become a tired old lady who preferred to sit alone at home by the fire.

2 Mr Williams, 46, was admitted to hospital after his wife had to call the police to their home. That day he had refused to get dressed and had been running around the house naked making unwanted sexual advances to his wife. His comments to her had been uncharacteristically coarse, harsh and threatening. When the police arrived he stood naked before them, shouted swear words at them and tried to sexually assault the woman police officer. In the preceding month he had lost his job as a bank manager because of some bad loan judgements he had made and some indiscrete comments to a female customer. His wife was bewildered and distraught because her husband of 20 years had always been such a mild-mannered and polite man. It was as if his whole character had changed.

3 Jemima, 26, a staff nurse, had three short-lived episodes of auditory hallucinations. Each episode had occurred when she was working a double shift at the nursing home she helped run. Each time she had been on duty for over 12 hours without rest or a food break. The voices she had heard were marked auditory hallucinations which had lasted for only a few minutes but had really frightened Jemima. Before these episodes she reported feeling faint for a few minutes and also experiencing the sensation of *déjà vu*.

MCQs

1 Recognised features of frontal lobe lesions include:
a perseveration
b disinhibition
c visual agnosia
d homonymous hemianopia
e receptive aphasia

2 Organic causes that may induce depressed mood include:
a hypothyroidism
b hyperthyroidism
c Cushing's disease
d bronchial carcinoma
e cerebrovascular accident

3 Dementia-like syndromes can be caused by:
a hypothyroidism
b vitamin B12 deficiency
c acute alcohol withdrawal
d neurosyphilis
e Huntington's chorea

Answers to cases

1 Hypothyroidism. Hypothyroidism is a reversible cause of dementia. Physical symptoms such as tiredness, constipation, mental and physical slowness and cold intolerance are suggestive of the illness.

2 Frontal lobe tumour. There are features of the frontal lobe syndrome — a description of personality change, coarsening of behaviour and disinhibition. Hypomania would be a reasonable differential diagnosis.

3 Temporal lobe epilepsy. There is a history of discrete short-lived psychotic episodes occurring when the patient is tired and possibly hypoglycaemic. *Déjà vu* is a common TLE symptom.

MCQ answers

1 a = T,   b = T,   c = F,   d = F,   e = F
2 All true
3 a = T,   b = T,   c = F,   d = T,   e = T

Explorations

The 'Further reading and references' section will help you to answer the following.

Links with medical history

1 Who was Phineas Gage? What horrific accident helped lead to the theory of cerebral localisation?

2 Who were Broca and Wernicke? What were their contributions to our understanding of speech? How did they make their discoveries and how did they analyse them?

3 What venereally transmitted infectious disease was responsible for many of the chronically mentally ill patients of the nineteenth century? What symptoms did they have and how was the neuropathology related to these symptoms?

Links with medicine

What are the main clinical features of systemic lupus

erythematosus (SLE)? What is the underlying pathology in SLE? How does the pathology link with the clinical features? What percentage of patients with SLE have psychiatric symptoms? How does the pathology of SLE link with these symptoms?

Links with genetics

What inherited condition may present with psychosis in middle age? How is it inherited? What can be done in terms of genetic counselling for relatives? How might relatives of the patient be affected by learning the results of predictive genetic testing?

Links with paediatrics

How common is schizophrenia in children? If you were to assess a 10-year-old boy who had a sudden onset of visual hallucinations and who had tried to fly out of a first floor window, what would you suspect as the cause? What questions would you ask the boy and the boy's parents?

Links with public health and epidemiology

1 What heavy metals can affect brain function? What public health initiatives aim to reduce the exposure of children to heavy metals?
2 Which causes of dementia are horizontally transmitted? How can transmission be prevented?

Links with neurology

During the physical examination of a patient what features on examination of the nervous system might suggest a cerebral lesion?

Links with psychology

What psychological tests might predict the presence of, and site of, brain lesions?

Further reading and references

Texts

ÁRNADÓTTIR G 1990 The brain and behaviour. Assessing cortical dysfunction through activities of daily living. C V Mosby & Co, St Louis

GLEITMAN H 1993 Psychology, 3rd edn. W W Norton & Co, New York

LINDESAY J, MACDONALD A, STARKE T 1990 Delirium in the elderly. Oxford University Press, Oxford

LISHMAN W A 1987 Organic psychiatry, 2nd edn. Oxford Medical Publications, Oxford

Papers

ADAMS F 1988 Emergency intravenous sedation of the delirious medically ill patient. Journal of Clinical Psychiatry 49 (suppl. 12): 22–26

Resources

Association to Combat Huntington's chorea,
108 Battersea High Street,
London SW11 3HP
Tel: 0171 223 7000

British Epilepsy Association,
Anstey House,
40 Hanover Square,
Leeds LS3 1BE
Tel: 01532 439393

British Migraine Association,
178a High Road,
Byfleet, Weybridge,
Surrey KT14 7ED.
Tel: 019323 52468

Link — The Neurofibromatosis Association,
120 London Road,
Kingston-upon-Thames,
Surrey KT2 6QJ
Tel: 0181 547 1636

Migraine Trust,
45 Great Ormond Street,
London WC1N 3HD
Tel: 0171 278 2676

Tourette Syndrome UK Association,
169 Wickham Street,
Welling,
Kent DA16 3BS
Tel: 0181 304 5446

The following organisations are dedicated to helping in HIV issues:

Avert,
PO Box 91,

Horsham,
West Sussex RH13 7YR
Tel: 01403 864010

Body Positive,
51b Philbeach Gardens,
London SW5 9EB
Tel: 0171 835 1045

Terence Higgins Trust,
BM Aida,
London WC1N 3XX
Tel: 0171 831 0330

Schizophrenia

Schizophrenia is often a chronic relapsing psychotic disorder that primarily affects thought and behaviour. It can be well controlled with antipsychotic drugs (sometimes called neuroleptics).

Contents

The onset of schizophrenia

CASE HISTORY 1

Jane was seen by a consultant on a domiciliary visit to the vicarage of St. Mary's church. Her father, the vicar, explained that Jane was a sixth form pupil at a local private school. She had always done well at school and had achieved high grades in her fifth form exams. She was hoping to go to university. Over the last few months, however, her behaviour had changed. She had started refusing to go to school but had declined to give any reason why. She spent her days writing in her room and had not eaten for the last 3 days. She would not let her parents in to see her and had barricaded the door. There was no history of drug abuse.

The consultant talked to her through the door and finally persuaded her to trust him sufficiently to let him in to her room. He found that Jane was a tall, thin girl with a pale face. The room smelt of urine and the walls had been covered in a fine, spidery writing. When the consultant tried to read what it said, she shouted at him. Jane looked at him suspiciously and, at times, seemed to be conferring with an unseen person as to how trustworthy the doctor was. The doctor could see scratch marks on her neck where Jane had cut herself with the blade of a pair of scissors. She said that this was 'to let the bad blood out'. Jane appeared alert and knew the time and date. When asked about her refusal to eat, Jane mumbled about her parents trying to poison her, because, she said, 'my mother offered me an Arrowroot Thin biscuit . . . that would make me thin . . . and she offered me some cabbage . . . that would turn me into a cabbage.'

The doctor felt that Jane's health was at risk because she had been harming and starving herself and that there was evidence of a mental disorder which warranted admission to hospital for further assessment.

What evidence is there that Jane is suffering from a psychotic disorder?

Firm evidence includes the asocial speech (muttering to unseen and unheard persons) which may

well mean she has auditory hallucinations and the concrete thoughts in her statement that eating Thin biscuits would make her thin and eating cabbage would turn her into a cabbage. Circumstantial evidence includes the social withdrawal, self-neglect, suspiciousness and marked alteration in her normal behaviour.

What evidence suggests that this is not an acute organic psychosis?

Jane is in clear consciousness (she alert and orientated). The onset of the illness is relatively insidious — her behaviour has changed over months, gradually becoming more bizarre and chaotic.

What are the diagnostic features of schizophrenia in this case?

Perceptual disorder (hallucinations) and thought disorder in clear consciousness, together with 'negative' symptoms of social withdrawal and significant and consistent change in her personal behaviour. Jane was a conscientious student but through illness has become self-absorbed and apathetic. Features of the illness have been present for months. Her suspiciousness of the consultant and her fear that she was being poisoned suggest a degree of paranoia. Hospital assessment would probe whether there were further persecutory delusions. Certainly there are enough grounds to make paranoid schizophrenia the primary differential diagnosis.

How would Jane be assessed in hospital?

The consultant might well suspect that his key differential diagnosis (paranoid schizophrenia) was correct but, because this is the first presentation of psychiatric illness in a young person, especial care must be taken to ensure that the diagnosis is correct. Organic illnesses can mimic schizophrenia and some have specific cures (such as hyperthyroidism and neurosyphilis or general paralysis of the insane). Reasonable care must be used to exclude these. Table 3.1 shows some other causes of schizophrenia-like illnesses.

Assessment would therefore include a full history and mental state examination, a physical exam-

Table 3.1   The differential diagnosis of schizophrenia

- Affective psychoses
- Schizoid personality
- Schizotypal personality
- Severe obsessional compulsive disorder
- Drug-induced psychosis
  (LSD, cannabis, ecstasy, cocaine, steroids etc)
- Thyrotoxicosis
- Cerebral tumour
- Temporal lobe epilepsy
- Huntington's chorea
- Cushing's disease
- Porphyria
- Hypothyroidism
- HIV — opportunistic cerebral infections
- Neurosyphilis

ination and various other investigations. Physical investigations would include a full blood count, urea and electrolytes, thyroid function tests, urine and blood drug screen and a screen for sexually transmitted diseases, specifically including syphilis. Besides blood tests, physical investigations should include an electroencephalogram (EEG) which would help identify any epileptic activity or focal lesions and some form of cerebral imaging (CT scan or MRI scan) to rule out cerebral lesions such as a prefrontal meningioma.

Why does schizophrenia often appear to begin in adolescence?

According to her father, Jane appears to have had a normal childhood and has always done well at school. The onset of schizophrenia at her age is a devastating event which may well disrupt her career and the rest of her life, but why should it arise now when her development to date has apparently been going so well?

Usually there is a prodromal phase to schizophrenia and people who later develop the illness are noticed to be unusual in their interests or absence of friends. Their premorbid personality is sometimes described as *schizoid* — aloof, cold, no friends, withdrawn, no sexual partners and with unusual religious or scientific interests. Jane appears to be different to this stereotype. Some research has suggested that even in such relatively

normal people there are 'soft' neurological signs present before the overt mental state features are noticed — slightly abnormal gaits in childhood, dysgraphaesthisia and proprioceptive errors. Current opinion is that schizophrenia originates perinatally from whatever cause (genetic and/or environmental), but classical schizophrenia only manifests later during adolescence or early adulthood.

Onset of schizophrenia — general points

- Schizophrenia mainly affects thought and behaviour as opposed to affect. It is often a chronic disorder in that there are multiple acute episodes and between these residual effects.
- The diagnosis of schizophrenia is usually made with the help of a longitudinal view of the patient, i.e. the form of the illness is as important as the content of the illness in making a diagnosis.
- Schizophrenia affects up to 1% of the population (up to 600 000 people in the UK). Given that it is often a chronically disabling condition it is, therefore, responsible for a great deal of the population's morbidity. It has an incidence of 18–20 cases per 100 000 population per year. Its peak age of onset differs for men and women. The average age of onset for men is 20–25 and the average age of onset for women is 25–30. In social terms chronic illnesses generally consume much of the total health budget. The cost of psychiatric health care has trebled in the last 20 years. In the United States schizophrenia consumes $35–40 billion per year in direct and indirect costs. In the UK, direct and indirect annual costs total £3.5 million.

Clinical features

Concepts of what schizophrenia actually is change with time. Different names and different criteria have been used to make the diagnosis at different times. This may be because the disease itself changes with time or because we are actually analysing a phenomenon with several different causes that all present a common picture, i.e. of disturbances of thought and behaviour. Prior to this century patients with general paralysis of the insane (GPI) caused by *Treponema pallidum* were classed in with schizophrenic-like patients. It may be that what we term schizophrenia today is a heterogenous disease with different causes.

The concept of schizophrenia

An illness like schizophrenia has been variously described over the years. Falvet in 1851 called it *folie circulaire*, Hecker in 1871 called it *hebephrenia*, Kahlbaum in 1874 described catatonia (a movement disorder) and *paranoia*. Kraepelin in 1878 pulled the various concepts together into one disease entity which he termed *dementia praecox* and said there were four types: simple, paranoid, hebephrenic and catatonic, depending on the clinical presentation. Simple dementia praecox involved a slow social decline, with apathy and withdrawal rather than florid psychotic symptoms. People with this typically became drifters or tramps. Paranoid dementia praecox involved fear and systematised persecutory delusions. The hebephrenic type was silly and facetious. Such terms enter common usage, with their meaning slightly shifted — hebephrenia was misappropriated by the public and corrupted to the phrase 'heebie-jeebies'. Catatonic patients were those with predominant motor symptoms — increased muscle tone, preservation of posture (patients could be manipulated like passive mannequins into unusual postures which they would maintain for hours), waxy flexibility and fear. Despite their persistent immobility such catatonic patients were acutely aware of their surroundings. Before suitable pharmacological treatments arrived, unless the catatonic episode aborted spontaneously, the patient would die through starvation or thirst unless carefully nursed.

Bleuler, in 1908, criticised the use of the term dementia praecox because he said that there was no global dementing process. He first used the term *schizophrenia* and said that there were four characteristics:

- Blunted **A**ffect
- Loosening of **A**ssociations
- **A**mbivalence
- **A**utism.

These characteristics were called the 'fours A's'. Blunted affect referred to a restricted range of affect. Loosening of associations referred to the thought

disorder present in schizophrenia. Ambivalence, or an inability to make decisions, was often seen in untreated cases where patients might hover for hours on the threshold of a doorway, uncertain whether to come in or go out (sometimes called ambitendence). Autism referred not to the childhood condition but to a retreat into an inner world, incomprehensible to the outsider.

The four diagnostic criteria of Bleuler have been revised over the years. Kurt Schneider listed the so-called 'first rank features' of schizophrenia in 1959. One of these, in the absence of organic disease, persistent affective disorder or drug intoxication, was sufficient for a diagnosis of schizophrenia:

- third person auditory hallucinations (running commentaries on the patient's actions or thoughts, or arguments about the patient)
- thought echo (echo de la pensée), thoughts spoken out loud (gedankenlautwerden)
- passivity phenomena (made actions, made emotions, made impulses)
- thought insertion, withdrawal, broadcasting
- delusional perception.

However, the criteria were criticised for being too narrow and only looking at a 'snapshot' of a patient at one point in time.

Current guidelines

The current guidelines used are those of ICD-10 from 1992:

A minimum requirement is one of the following symptoms: thought echo, insertion, withdrawal, broadcasting, passivity phenomena, delusional perception, third person hallucinations and persistent delusions — all in clear consciousness.

Other symptoms used to make the diagnosis (two must be present) include persistent hallucinations in any modality, thought blocking, thought disorder, catatonic behaviour, negative symptoms, loss of social function.

Symptoms should have been present for at least one month. This emphasis on the *form* of the illness helps exclude patients with transient psychotic symptoms or signs. Affective disorder should have been excluded. Symptoms should be present in the absence of overt brain disease, drug use or epilepsy (which can all mimic schizophrenia). ICD-10 lists the following types: paranoid, hebephrenic, catatonic, residual (a chronic state) and simple.

CASE HISTORY 2

J. Albert Arthur Andrew Churchill Chamberlain was a man who went under several aliases and had a career as a small time con-man. Some days he was Albert Chamberlain and some days he was Andrew Churchill.

He presented to his general practitioner with feelings of 'great sadness and loss of sincerity' as he put it. His general practitioner found his speech difficult to understand, but understood that his main concerns seemed to be about his ex-wife. He claimed that his ex-wife was plotting with the British Security Forces to remove his 'sincerity and personality'. The GP noted down some of his speech verbatim: 'My divorced wife has an albigisty of conscience which she has terpolated with the Security Forces. They're debating my existence even now. They're saying we will drain his face of emotions, put our emotions into him and alter what the doctor's writing on the page to alter the circumstance and the circumcision of the truth.'

On further questioning the patient seemed wholly convinced that a transmitter had been inserted into his neck — he said he could actually feel it there — and that the transmitter was designed to put his wife's thoughts into his head. He could distinctly hear conversations between his wife and agents of the British Security Forces commenting on his thoughts and actions.

What Schneiderian first rank features does this patient exhibit?

He clearly describes a multiple third person auditory hallucination giving a running commentary on his thoughts and actions (his wife and agents of the British Security Forces). In addition, his wife's thoughts are inserted into his mind (thought insertion) and he feels that his emotions are being replaced by those of another (made emotions — a passivity phenomenon).

What is the significance of his using words like 'albigisty' and 'terpolated'?

These are examples of *neologisms* embedded here in thought disordered speech. Neologisms are sometimes a feature of schizophrenic thought disorder, although neologisms are not pathognomonic of schizophrenia.

What kind of schizophrenia is this?

In view of the persecutory delusions which have been elaborated into a delusional system it would seem that Mr Chamberlain has paranoid schizophrenia.

CASE HISTORY 3

Shakil, 32, was brought to casualty by his brother who had found him by accident in a nearby seaside town. Shakil had been missing from home for several years. By chance his brother had seen Shakil walking down the road and had followed him home. Home had turned out to be ramshackle flat above an empty sewing machine shop.

His brother had been disgusted to find the remains of Shakil's last meal, an unplucked, ungutted and uncooked pigeon. Shakil said he had put the bird in the oven for half-an-hour to cook it, but since the electricity supply had been long since discontinued, the attempt had been pointless.

Shakil had been unwilling to draw unemployment benefit because he said the money should be sent to the Third World instead. A god, called Abu-Lafram, who lived in the bathroom, had told Shakil that he should deny himself for the benefit of the Third World. Shakil had little furniture left, he had sold most of it to buy bread and aluminium tin foil. He had used the tin foil to line the walls of the flat to protect Abu-Lafram from the evils of Western civilisation that seeped through the walls. His brother had been most upset when he had told Shakil the bad news that his mother had died whilst Shakil had been away from home. Shakil had started to laugh.

On interview in casualty Shakil was unkempt and dressed in a grimy boiler suit to which blood and feathers adhered. A large pentagram was daubed on the breast pocket. Shakil giggled at times and appeared to be listening to some voice other people could not hear. He was mildly thought disordered and easily distracted, pacing about casualty, preaching the gospel of Abu-Lafram to other patients and using various neologisms. When he was asked how he felt about the death of his mother, Shakil grinned and said that his mother was a 'white cloud in a darkening and prejudiced sky'. He claimed to be a prophet of Abu-Lafram and that he had been chosen as his first earthly disciple. Abu-Lafram talked to him throughout the day in a sonorous male voice, 'realer than the realest reality'. The thoughts he had had since knowing Abu-Lafram were 'the purest of purée' and were broadcast out of Shakil's head by Abu-Lafram for 'the benefit of all mankind'. Shakil did not believe that he was ill, but was adamant that he was a 'chosen one'.

What evidence is there to support a diagnosis of schizophrenia?

There is a history of declining social functioning and withdrawal. Shakil is observed to be hallucinated and says that he hears the voice of Abu-Lafram, a god, who talks only to him (second person auditory hallucination). Shakil has a variety of secondary delusions based on this hallucinatory voice — that he is the chosen one and a prophet. The delusions have a markedly grandiose flavour. Shakil also has an inappropriate affect (laughing when first told of his mother's death). There is a complete lack of insight into his condition — he is able to live with the apparent paradox of being a 'chosen one' and living in squalor.

What is the relevance of the patient's lack of insight?

If Shakil does not accept that he is ill he will be less likely to accept hospital treatment. There is good evidence that, without treatment, his lifestyle alone is likely to lead to damage to his health. Compulsory admission and treatment may be necessary.

The course of the illness

The onset in men is earlier than in women (20–25 and 25–30 respectively). Before the illness can be recognised there is often a prodromal phase in the late teenage years with social isolation, interest in fringe cults, social withdrawal (e.g. living alone in their bedroom with minimal contact with family) and no friends. Patients with schizophrenia often have 'neurological soft signs' — dysgraphaesthesia, clumsiness, movement disorders and the like. Recent research has indicated that such soft signs, dyskinesias and gait disturbances may be detectable in childhood before the onset of florid psychotic symptoms. Home movies of American children who later developed schizophrenia have been investigated and compared with home movies of children who have not developed the disease in later life. The movies were rated by neurologists 'blind' to the subsequent diagnosis. The presence of such a 'soft-sign' in childhood is not pathognomonic of schizophrenia but such signs are seen significantly more often in children at risk for schizophrenia. Therefore, symptoms and signs may predate (by many years) the next phase, which is the 'active' phase of the illness, characterised by positive symptoms such as hallucinations, delusions, thought insertion and the like. The active phase coincides with the 'obvious' onset of the illness. Table 3.2 shows positive and negative features of schizophrenia.

The active phase may last forever if untreated or may resolve spontaneously without treatment (although this would be very rare). Most active phases can be aborted by antipsychotic medication. After an active episode of schizophrenia there may be a complete return to normal function and no further episode may happen. It is more likely that there will be several episodes through life and that function and personality may be damaged. This impairment of function/personality may be progressive. Often the active phase with its positive features is replaced by a residual phase characterised by 'negative' features such as blunted affect or poverty of thought.

What happens to people in the years after a first episode of schizophrenia? About 20% of patients have only one episode and had no impairment

Table 3.2 Positive and negative feature of schizophrenia

Positive features	Negative features
Hallucinations • second person auditory 75% • third person auditory 58% • visual 49%	Affective blunting 96%
Delusions • persecutory 81% • religious 31% • grandiose 35% • of reference 49%	Alogia (impoverished thinking) 53%
Bizarre behaviour • clothing 20% • sexual 33%	Avolition/apathy 95%
Formal thought disorder 50% Thought dysfunction • broadcasting 23% • insertion 33% • withdrawal 27%	Anhedonia/asociality • few interests 95% • little sexual interest 69% • few friends 96%

of function or personality. Thirty-five per cent go on to have several episodes with no impairment between. About 10% have multiple episodes of schizophrenia with a static level of functional and personality impairment between. Thirty-five per cent have mutiple episodes with increasing levels of impairment between as in Figure 3.1.

In a study which looked at the 35 year outcome of schizophrenia, 20% of those with a first episode in the 1940s were well while 45% were incapacitated by their illness. Sixty-seven per cent had never married and 58% had never worked since their first episode.

One-sixth of people with schizophrenia die by their own hand, often in response to psychotic symptoms, e.g. second person auditory hallucinations telling them to kill themselves.

Features which predispose to a bad prognosis in schizophrenia

- Insidious onset
- Neurological soft signs

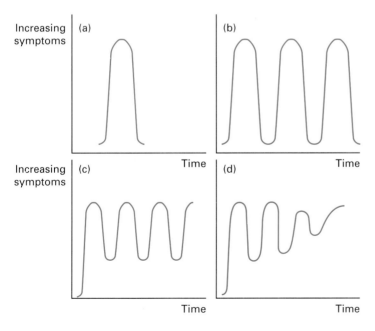

Fig. 3.1 The course of schizophrenia over time. a) patients with only one episode 20%; b) patients with several episodes with no impairment between 35%; c) patients with multiple episodes with some static level of impairment between 10%; and d) patients with multiple episodes and increasing.

- Past psychiatric history
- History of violence
- Long duration of first illness
- Emotional blunting
- Social withdrawal
- Poor psychosexual functioning.

In summary, a minority of a fifth of patients with

a first episode of schizophrenia have a good prognosis. The majority have multiple episodes and about half have chronic impairment of function affecting their ability to form relationships and work. Schizophrenia can, therefore, be seen as a chronically disabling disorder with important family and social consequences.

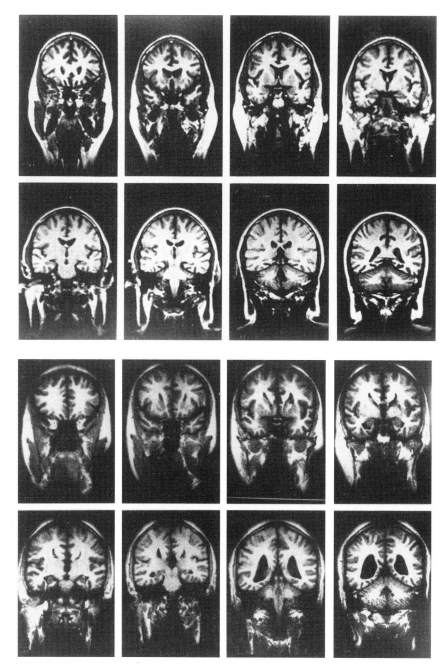

Fig. 3.2 Control MRI scans of a normal brain.

Fig. 3.3 MRI scans of the brain of a patient with schizophrenia showing enlarged ventricles and callosal agenesis.

Aetiology

Kraepelin delineated 'functional psychoses' from 'organic psychoses'. Organic psychoses included dementias and epilepsy. Kraepelin was well aware of the pathology of the brain in such illnesses. The brain, however, looked normal in post-mortems of affective and schizophrenia sufferers. Hence Kraepelin called affective disorder and schizophrenia 'functional psychoses', implying that there was no gross pathology to be seen in the brain. Modern neuroimaging has however found an organic basis for some affective and schizophrenic disorders (Figs 3.2, 3.3, 3.4 & 3.5) and so the term 'functional psychosis' is no longer used.

For a long time, when schizophrenia was seen as a 'functional' disorder, there were doctors who advocated that the whole concept of schizophrenia was untrustworthy and not an illness but a sociological phenomenon, i.e. that patients with schizophrenia were normal people driven insane by an insane world. Some pointed to the role of the mother and said that some mothers' rearing behaviours were 'schizophrenogenic', i.e. that the mothers brought up their children incorrectly and induced schizophrenic thought patterns in them. They did this by using a 'double bind' e.g. asking the child to do something, but giving a contrary non-verbal message. Other doctors and psychologists suggested that mental illness was a 'myth'.

The efficacy of antipsychotic drugs and recent advances in biological research have countered this 1970s concept but difficulties with the concept of schizophrenia remain. It is possible that the people who have schizophrenia are a heterogenous group with different areas of their brains affected to varying degrees by neurochemical imbalances, neurodevelopmental problems, genetic defects, viral infections or perinatal damage amongst other causes. Continuing research is essential. A treatable cause for a percentage of patients is worth hunting for. Prior to this century, between 10 and 30% of schizophrenia-like patients probably had neurosyphilis. Without the knowledge of neurosyphilis that we now have, this group of treatable patients would merely be a sub-group of an even larger population of undifferentiated schizophrenia.

Families and schizophrenia

Genetic aspects

If one family member has schizophrenia, the closer you are to that individual in genetic terms, the more likely you are to get schizophrenia too. In twin studies, if one twin of a dizygotic pair gets schizophrenia (the case is called 'the proband'), the other twin has a 14% chance of also getting schizophrenia in his or her lifetime (lifetime risk). In a monozygotic pair the twin of the proband has a 50% lifetime risk. This shows that the higher the proportion of genetic

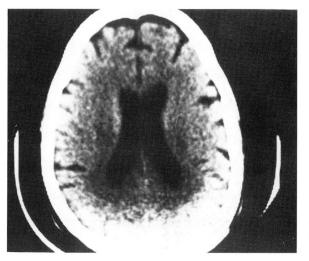

Fig. 3.4 MRI scan of the brain of a patient with schizophrenia showing enlarged lateral ventricles and cortical thinning.

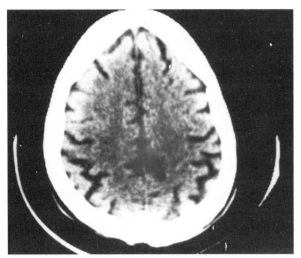

Fig. 3.5   MRI scan of the brain of a patient with schizophrenia showing widened cortical sulci.

Table 3.3   Lifetime risks of developing schizophrenia.

• Member of the general public	1%
• Children who have one parent with schizophrenia	12%
• Children of parents who both have schizophrenia	46%
• Siblings of a patient with schizophrenia	8–14%
• Parents of a patient with schizophrenia	5–10%
• Second degree relatives of patient with schizophrenia	2.5%

material in common the greater the chance of developing schizophrenia. Table 3.3 shows the lifetime risks of developing schizophrenia for different individuals.

Spectrum disorder

Relatives of patients with schizophrenia have been noted to have mild features of the illness themselves to a certain degree. They may have some mild loosening of associations in their everyday speech but not to such a degree that it could be described as thought disorder. This has resulted in the idea that schizophrenia may be one extreme of a spectrum of schizophrenia-related disorders including language disturbance and personality differences such as schizoid or eccentric behaviour.

The family environment

The emphasis on community care has meant that instead of sufferers being removed to large asylums for most of their lives, they can be accommodated in the community within a family setting. There are advantages and disadvantages for the sufferer and the family. Some research has indicated that certain types of family environment may be harmful to the patient but that characteristics of this environment can be altered with help to enable the individual to remain within the family. The environment which promoted a greater frequency of relapses is called a *high expressed emotion environment*. High EE environments involve a lot of negative criticism towards the patient, over-involvement by certain members of the family, expressed hostility and greater than 35 hours per week face-to-face contact. Education programmes for the family seek to explain features of the illness to the family, reduce the amount of hostile criticism and 'ration' contact. Such programmes have been shown to reduce EE and relapse rates.

Organic evidence for schizophrenia

Table 3.4 outlines some of the current biological evidence for a physical basis for schizophrenia. Current opinion favours an organic aetiology based

Table 3.4   Evidence of a physical basis for schizophrenia

Family and twin studies

EEG abnormalities
• abnormal theta and delta waves

Neurological soft signs (in 75% of patients)

PET scanning
• reduced glucose metabolism in frontal lobes (so-called hypofrontality responsible for negative symptoms)

CT/NMR scanning
• cortical thinning
• lateral ventricular enlargement
• sulcal enlargement
• cerebellar atrophy
• reduction in temporal lobe and hippocampal volume
(Abnormalities almost exclusively in early onset young men)

on the neurodevelopmental hypothesis. According to this hypothesis, an early brain insult affects brain development leading to abnormalities which are expressed in the mature brain. There are animal precedents for such delayed effects. If the satiety centre of the rat hypothalamus is experimentally damaged in rat neonates no effect can be discerned on eating behaviour until day 40, when rats become anorexic. The onset of the anorexia seems to coincide with rat adolescence. Similarly, if small areas in the ape frontal lobe are experimentally damaged no effect on behaviour can be discerned until age 8 when the ape begins its adolescence. It is argued from these animal models that it is possible that in schizophrenia the effects of the pre- or perinatal insult lie dormant until late adolescence and the onset of positive symptoms. Some people have proposed that these perinatal insults involve hypoxia or birth trauma. Others have suggested that maternal viral infections damage the developing brain in utero.

Some schizophrenia family pedigrees have recently been linked to markers on chromosome 5, but this work has been refuted.

Treatment

CASE HISTORY 4

Michael and his father were brought to casualty by the police. Michael had tried to set light to his father's bedroom. When his father had smelt smoke and tried to stop his son, Michael had hit him with a table lamp. Whilst his father was having his wounds tended by the accident and emergency doctor a psychiatrist was called to see Michael. Michael was so disturbed that it took three policemen to keep him in casualty. He shouted that the devil was after him and that the policemen were demons.

The psychiatrist who saw him noted that Michael was in his early twenties and dishevelled in appearance. There were smuts over his face from the fire he had tried to light. She was only able to speak to him briefly. He was very frightened that he would be killed by the police and had auditory and visual hallucinations. He was responding to 'the angel of death' which he said was standing in the corner of the room. The psy-

chiatrist checked that he was in clear consciousness and asked whether Michael had been taking any street drugs. It seemed that he was grossly orientated and that he had not been abusing drugs (according to Michael and his father). Although he could respond to closed questions, his answers became more thought disordered if he was allowed to continue. Once he referred to the devil putting 'demon thoughts' into his head.

Michael was so disturbed that a detailed history was impossible. Shortly after the psychiatrist arrived to see him, Michael lashed out at her with his fists saying that the angel had told him she was the 'whore of Babylon'. He was desperately trying to wriggle free of the policemen's grasp in order to leave the accident and emergency department.

What is the differential diagnosis?

Michael's presentation is marked by fear and he has various persecutory hallucinations and secondary delusions. He acts on these fearsome hallucinations. For instance, he tries to attack the psychiatrist because a voice tells him she is the 'whore of Babylon'. There is no doubt that this is a psychotic illness, but what is the cause? If the illness was of a very sudden onset, with a previously 'normal' premorbid personality, then an acute organic psychosis due to drugs might be top of the differential diagnosis in a young man. Drugs like ecstasy, cocaine and amphetamines may all lead to such an acute presentation. However, if the illness had a more insidious onset (days or weeks), then paranoid schizophrenia would be a likely candidate. It is worth bearing in mind that Michael and his father deny any drug history and that Michael seems orientated. If there was no drug history and he was in clear consciousness, then paranoid schizophrenia would be the main diagnosis. However, it is possible for drug users to deny their habit and Michael would need further assessment (full history, physical examination and investigations including a drug screen) before a final diagnosis could be made.

How could Michael be managed?

Michael presents a management problem. He is not in hospital voluntarily, he has allegedly assaulted his father and allegedly tried to set a fire. There are two immediate problems: firstly, he is mentally disordered and violent; and secondly, he is not giving consent to remain and be treated so that there are legal issues to be dealt with. There is a clear requirement for emergency sedation so that the psychiatrist can gain control of the situation. Mental Health legislation or common law usually provides for a one-off emergency treatment. To sedate a young, highly aroused male safely would require an adequate dose of an antipsychotic such as chlorpromazine or droperidol given via a suitable route. Oral medication may be too slow in this situation and an intramuscular injection might be required. An example might be 100 mg chlorpromazine i.m. Intravenous chlorpromazine could promote a dangerous arrhythmia and kill the patient. *Intravenous* sedation with benzodiazepines might be an adjunct for quick control, e.g. diazepam 5–10 mg given via a slow intravenous injection. However, attempting to find a vein in a writhing patient can be an impossible and hazardous task. It is important from a safety point of view to have adequate numbers of people restraining the individual before, during and after the injection is given. It may take some time before the intramuscular injection of chlorpromazine works. Such restraint should not be excessive and must avoid damage to chest or abdomen.

Mental health legislation usually covers cases where mentally disordered people are removed by the police from private property or public places to what is termed a 'place of safety' such as casualty or a police station. To admit him to hospital for assessment, however, may require further legal steps.

┤ CASE HISTORY 5 ├────────────

Julian is 35, lives with his mother and attends a drop-in centre run by a local mental health charity. He was diagnosed as having schizophrenia 10 years ago and has been hospitalised five times for exacerbations of his illness. He has been on various treatments but has not found any that remove all his symptoms. He always complains of a voice that tells him to do various things. Sometimes the voice asks him to do embarrassing things like drop his trousers in public and other times the voice becomes quite threatening, telling him to jump off a motorway bridge into the traffic below. He has been unemployed for 10 years, has few friends (except other attenders at the drop-in centre) and has never had a girl friend. He spends long periods in his room, lying on his bed smoking or sleeping. He complains that he never feels happy and never feels sad. Recently he has been resisting the voice telling him to stop taking his chlorpromazine tablets. He usually takes 200 mg chlorpromazine three times a day, with 5 mg of procyclidine twice a day. He resists the voice for so long and then usually does stop taking his medication and as a consequence relapses

---

How is chlorpromazine metabolised?

Chlorpromazine is metabolised by the liver. There is a substantial first-pass metabolism so that almost 80% of the oral dose is removed before entering the general circulation. Liver enzymes become induced over time and so proportionately less drug reaches the CNS (see the section on 'Physical treatments' for further information on antipsychotic drugs).

What is the function of procyclidine?

Procyclidine is an example of an anticholinergic, often prescribed with antipsychotics to overcome acute movement disorders like dystonia and other cholinergic side-effects. Such anticholinergics should not be prescribed automatically with antipsychotics but on a more rationalised basis.

What negative features of schizophrenia does Julian have?

Social withdrawal, hyposexuality, blunted affect and apathy.

How else might Julian be managed?

Julian's symptoms conflict with his treatment in that his hallucinations affect his compliance — he has to constantly resist a voice telling him to stop taking his tablets. The exacerbations of schizophrenia which occur when he stops his maintenance treatment of chlorpromazine are unpleasant and potentially avoidable. If Julian would agree to regular injections of depot antipsychotics (e.g. flupen-thixol 40 mg every fortnight), these would relieve him of the burden of constantly having to remember to take his tablets and would enable the community nurse who gives the injections to monitor his mental state and compliance.

Another way of looking at the problem might be to say that Julian still has untreated positive and negative symptoms of his schizophrenia. These seem to be resistant to conventional treatments. If an alternative could be found that effectively removed the auditory hallucinations then perhaps compliance would not be a problem. About 20% of schizophrenia proves to be resistant like this. A proportion of these resistant cases may respond to an atypical antipsychotic called clozapine. Clozapine might occasionally be used as an alternative to traditional antipsychotic agents because of its different mode of action. Clozapine is not available as a depot injection. It can produce white blood cell dyscrasias so the blood count must be very carefully monitored. Despite the risk of dyscrasia in about 1% of clozapine treated patients, the benefit of treatment may outweigh the potential risk.

Services for schizophrenia

Entry to services

Initial diagnosis is either by the psychiatrist who may become involved when the patient first presents to casualty, by out-patient referral from the GP, through domiciliary consultation requests from the GP for an assessment in the patient's home or by calls to police stations to assess people in the police cells. Diagnosis must rule out treatable organic causes, e.g. temporal lobe epilepsy and other organic causes, e.g. Huntington's chorea and drug-induced psychosis. Assessment includes family, psychological and social assessments and corroborative histories.

Initial service options

Cases can be managed in the community with sufficient out-patient resources such as a clinic, day hospital and community psychiatric nurse (CPN) support. This is possible when the diagnosis is clear-cut and where the illness is 'mild'.

In cases where there is loss of insight, refusal of treatment and perhaps violent behaviour (based on, say, delusions or hallucinations) towards the self or others, then in-patient assessment or treatment is required. If consent to admission is not forthcoming, then, depending on the circumstances, use of mental health legislation may be needed.

Treatment can begin once a firm diagnosis is made, with a move to maintenance treatment with i.m. depot injections as an option. In-patient and day hospital stays might be from a few weeks to a year.

Medium-term service options

Patients in remission can be managed in the community or with day hospital backup. Patients may attend a variety of voluntary and state support services designed to rehabilitate them. Such facilities include social service drop-in centres, MIND day centres and clinics. CPN support and computer follow-up to monitor and give treatment is essential to prevent patients 'falling through the net'.

Long-term service options

If relapse occurs, rapid treatment responses in clinic may prevent a further in-patient stay. Further episodes may require readmission to the day hospital or in-patient facilities. Once the episode is under control, return to the community can be renegotiated. Persistent psychosis may require altered treatment strategies, e.g. with clozapine, or admission to dedicated rehabilitation wards. There will always be a need for long-term hospitalisation in a minority of cases.

Dedicated sheltered housing is sometimes available through the Richmond Fellowship, MIND, social services and other agencies.

Most cases can be adequately managed in the community, usually in their own homes by liaison between CPNs, GPs, psychiatrists and social services.

Self-assessment

MCQs

1 Features associated with a good prognosis in a first episode of schizophrenia include:

a astereognosis
b poor psychosexual functioning
c sudden onset of symptoms
d emotional blunting
e social withdrawal

2 Antipsychotic drugs include:
a benperidol
b sulpiride
c risperidone
d flupenthixol
e dexamphetamine

3 Positive features of schizophrenia include:
a anhedonia
b avolition
c thought disorder
d visual hallucinations
e delusions of reference

Short answer questions

1 List the first rank features of schizophrenia.
2 What are neurological soft signs?
3 What agencies contribute to the care of schizophrenia in the community?
4 What investigations would you use to assess a patient presenting with auditory hallucinations and why?

MCQ answers

1 a = F, b = F, c = T, d = F, e = F
2 a = T, b = T, c = T, d = T, e = F
3 a = F, b = F, c = T, d = T, e = T

Explorations

Links with neurology and neuroanatomy

What tests can be done in a neurological examination to detect 'soft signs' such as dysgraphaesthesia? What is the neuroanatomical basis of such soft signs? What is 'cerebral localisation'? What links can you establish between symptoms in schizophrenia and the possible site of brain pathology? For instance, where might problems such as thought disorder be located in the brain?

Links with pharmacology

How are antipsychotic drugs metabolised? What different neurotransmitter systems do the drugs chlorpromazine and clozapine act upon?

Links with obstetrics and gynaecology

What evidence is there to link birth trauma, perinatal brain damage and schizophrenia? How good is that evidence?

LEARNING POINTS

Schizophrenia

- A minority of patients suffer a single episode of the illness.
- First line treatments involve dopamine (D2) receptor blockers.
- Long-term treatment with antipsychotic depot injections helps prevent relapse.
- The aetiology of schizophrenia is unknown, but there is evidence for an early neurodevelopmental abnormality.
- In a significant minority of patients MRI scans show brain abnormalities.
- In diagnosing schizophrenia doctors should exclude other causes of psychosis such as epilepsy.

Further reading and references

Texts

GELDER M, GATH D, MAYOU R 1989 Schizophrenia and schizophrenia-like disorders. In: Oxford Textbook of Psychiatry. Oxford Medical Publications, Oxford, pp 268–323

KENDELL R E, ZEALLEY A K 1993 Schizophrenia. In: Companion to Psychiatric Studies, 5th edn. Churchill Livingstone, Edinburgh, pp 397–426

SIMS A 1988 Disorders of the thinking process. In: Symptoms in the Mind. Baillière Tindall, Oxford, pp 105–125

Papers

ANDREASEN N 1990 Magnetic resonance imaging of the brain in schizophrenia. Archives of General Psychiatry, 47: 35–44

MCNEIL T F, HARTY B, BENNOW G et al. 1993 Neuromotor deviation in offspring of psychotic mothers: a selective developmental deficiency in two groups of children at heightened psychiatric risk? Journal of Psychiatric Research 27(21): 39–54

MURRAY R M, JONES P, O'CALLAGHAN E et al. 1992 Genes, viruses and neurodevelopmental schizophrenia. Journal of Psychiatric Research 26(4): 225–35

SHEPHERD M, WATT D, FALLOON I et al. 1989 The natural history of schizophrenia: a five-year follow-up study of outcome and prediction in a representative sample of schizophrenics. Psychological Medicine Suppl. 15, 46

TSUANG M T, WOOLSON R F, FLEMING J A 1979 Long-term outcome of major psychoses. Archives of General Psychiatry 36: 1295

VAUGHN C E, LEFF J P 1976 Influence of family and social factors on the course of psychiatric illness. British Journal of Psychiatry 129: 125

Schizophrenia in literature

BARNES M, BERKE J 1971 Mary Barnes. Two Accounts of a Journey through Madness.

KESEY K 1962 One Flew over the Cuckoo's Nest.

SCOTT FITZGERALD F 1934 Tender is the Night

Resources

National Schizophrenia Fellowship,
28 Castle Street,
Kingston-upon-Thames KT1 1SS
Tel: 0181 547 3937

Richmond Fellowship,
8 Addison Road,
London W14 8DL
Tel: 0171 603 6373

SANE — Schizophrenia: A National Emergency,
2nd Floor,
199–205 Old Marylebone Road,
London NW1 5QP
Tel: 0171 724 6520

MIND,
Mental Health Foundation
8, Hallam Street,
London WC1N 6DH.

Affective disorders

Affective disorders are predominantly disturbances of mood that are severe in nature and persistent despite the influence of external events.

Contents

Classification

Everybody's mood varies according to events in the world around them. We are happy when we achieve something or when we are enjoying a friend's company. We are saddened when we fail a test or lose something. When people are sad they sometimes say that they are 'depressed', but the clinical depressions that are seen by doctors differ from the low mood brought on by everyday setbacks. Clinically important disturbances of mood are known as *affective disorders* (or mood disorders). Affective disorders are more severe and more persistent than simple sadness.

Our normal emotions of happiness and sadness can become polarised into more severe forms. Happiness can become elation or mania and sadness can become profound despair or depression. This polarisation can be called a *bipole*, with mania at one extreme and depression at the other.

Patients who suffer with repeated episodes of depression have recurrent depressive disorder. When patients suffer manic episodes and depressive episodes they are said to have bipolar affective disorder (Figure 4.1).

Depressive episodes can be classified into mild, moderate and severe types with or without psychotic symptoms.

A condition where the mood is peristently low, but which does not quite fulfil all the criteria for a depressive episode, is sometimes called *dysthymia*.

Major depression is relatively common. Community studies have found prevalence rates of between 5 and 20%. About 10% of people over 65 have a major depressive episode at any one time. The incidence of depression seems to be higher in women than men and in urban rather than rural settings. Figure 4.2 shows how many cases of depression there are in a small general practice of 3000 patients. You can also see how many of these illnesses are detected by family doctors and how many are treated by psychiatrists.

Depression

Presentation

General

Depression is often accompanied by slowing of thought and *biological features of depression* altogether unlike everyday sadness (Table 4.1).

Crying is a frequent symptom, although some individuals are reluctant to admit this, and others feel so depressed it is as if they have 'gone beyond crying'.

Suicidal ideation

Suicidal ideas occur in most depressed people and asking about these is a crucial aspect of their assessment. Depressed patients often find it a relief to talk about these ideas with their doctor. Asking about

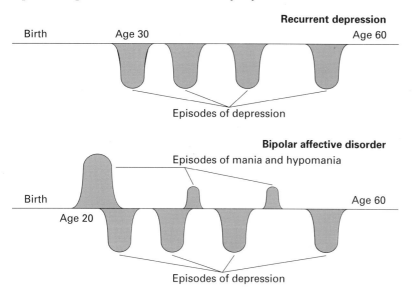

Fig. 4.1   The lifetime course of affective disorders

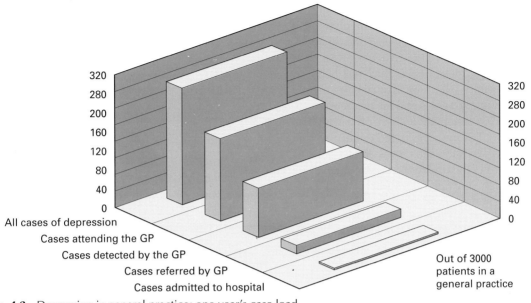

Fig. 4.2 Depression in general practice: one year's case load

---

Table 4.1 Biological features of depression
• Sleep disturbance (most importantly early morning wakening)
• Loss of appetite (also known as anorexia)
• Weight loss
• Diurnal mood variation (perhaps feeling sad and slow in the morning and brightening through the day)
• Constipation
• Reduced sexual drive (loss of libido)
• Psychomotor retardation (slowing of thoughts and actions)

suicidal ideas is a sequential process, beginning with questions about the severity of the low mood, then asking about if the patient has ever felt that life is not worth living, following this by enquiring whether the patient has ever felt like ending their own life, and finally assessing whether the patient has any particular plans in mind.

Appearance

On mental state examination depressed patients may appear unkempt or untidy. Depressed people feel bad about themselves and also lack the motivation to care for their appearance. The normally appearance conscious person may have stopped combing their hair and washing as often as before. Women may stop using make-up and men may stop shaving. When you interview someone who is depressed they may sit dejectedly, gazing down at the floor. You may notice that they do not make eye contact with you and that they fail to smile in response to greetings and jokes and are preoccupied and serious in manner. Their movements may be minimal or slowed to such an extent that they are prepared to sit alone brooding in a chair or lying in bed for hours during the day. They may appear unusually thin, having lost weight because of poor appetite. Occasionally the typical picture of psychomotor retardation may be replaced by a restless agitation and distraught displays of weeping.

Their speech may be minimal and monosyllabic or they may even be mute. Depressed speech lacks spontaneity and variety and may be spoken in a monotone. The facial expression may show sadness, anxiety or sometimes a masklike absence of emotion described as flattened affect.

Mental state

When you ask about thoughts and preoccupations the depressed patient may describe a catalogue of worries about money, close relationships or the health of themselves or others. Rarely they may say that there are almost no thoughts in their head because their thoughts have slowed down so much. Depressed people think little of themselves, their abilities or their achievements. They feel helpless, hopeless and guilty over past misdemeanours and that the world is a bad place and the future is exceptionally bleak. Occasionally depression becomes so severe that it takes on a psychotic quality so that hallucinations and delusions, consistent with low mood, manifest themselves. Hallucinations are characteristically unpleasant. Auditory hallucinations, usually in the second person, are derogatory, e.g. 'you're a fat cow!', 'you're so evil you should be put to death'. Auditory hallucinations are more common than hallucinations in other modalities. Sometimes olfactory hallucinations occur, e.g. a patient smelling rotting flesh, but such hallucinations may suggest an underlying organic cause such as a frontal lobe tumour which should be excluded. Abnormal sensory experiences are rare, however, and it is more usual for sensory experiences to be diminished, if anything, so that the world becomes grey and unpleasantly quiet and food seems uncharacteristically bland.

If present, delusions are usually secondary to low self-esteem, guilt, anxiety, fear or hallucinations. Delusions of guilt are sometimes extreme: 'I am responsible for the AIDS epidemic'. Delusions of ill health, sometimes called hypochondriacal delusions, may involve a conviction that the individual is riddled with cancer when there is no objective evidence of carcinoma. Often there is a theme of deserved punishment to such delusions: 'My face is rotting away with venereal disease because of what I did when I was young'. An extreme bodily delusion is the *nihilistic* delusion, e.g. 'I have no bowels' or 'My head is emptied of its brains'. Delusions of poverty and infestation are other examples of depressive delusions. Cognitive testing is often problematic. Depressed people find concentration particularly difficult and, although they are grossly orientated to time, place and person, tests of attention (such as serial sevens and the months of the year reversed) are poorly performed. Memory testing may suggest a short-term memory defect but the apparently poor memory is often due to problems with registration and concentration rather than recall. Depression in the elderly can mimic

dementia. This kind of problem is called a *pseudo-dementia*, and the apparent memory defect usually resolves once the depression has been treated.

┌─ CASE HISTORY 1 ├──────────────────

Janet Gordon was 35 when she lost her job as a manageress of a department store. At first she looked on her period of unemployment as an opportunity to try out activities she had not had time for before. She went hillwalking and painting every day. Two months later she had lost interest in these things and was convinced that she would never work again, although she had an exemplary work record. Her sleep at night was poor and she had started going to bed during the day. Janet cried almost daily and had lost interest in the food she cooked. All food tasted bland, she told her mother (who was concerned when she saw how much weight Janet had lost). At her mother's suggestion Janet went to her family doctor where she complained about how tired she always felt and asked for some sleeping tablets to help her sleep at night.

What biological features of depression are present?

Two clear features are Janet's lack of appetite (anorexia) and weight loss. We are told that her sleep was poor but we need to know exactly what the sleep problem was before we can say whether this was early morning wakening.

What precipitated the depression?

Adverse life events such as exam failure, bereavement and job loss may precede the onset of depression. In Janet's case the onset of depression is gradual, coming on some weeks after the loss of her job. Sometimes the onset of depression is so gradual that it is difficult for the depressed individual to date exactly when the illness started. It is as if the depression has crept up on them, in which case it may only be apparent to others. Because the depression has become a way of life to the depressed person only outsiders can see the illness for what it is. In Janet's case it is her mother who asks her to seek help.

How does Janet present her problem to her doctor?

Some people are wary of taking psychological symptoms to their doctor. They know that some-thing is wrong with them but consciously or uncon-sciously choose to take the symptoms that they feel doctors will be most interested in. Janet chooses to present her fatigue as her main problem and asks for sleeping tablets. Other depressed people will take bodily symptoms of anxiety and depres-sion to their doctor — headaches, muscular aches and pains, tremors and palpitations for instance. Depressed people may be very concerned about their health and seek multiple physical investiga-tions because they are sure there is some morbid physical cause for the wretched way they feel. In these cases the doctor must be very certain that there is no underlying physical problem before dismiss-ing the depressed individual's concerns. It is possi-ble for people to be depressed and physically ill. It is well documented that about one-quarter of medical in-patients have some depressive symptoms.

CASE HISTORY 2

Alan Benson was brought to the accident and emergency department by his son. Alan had tried to hang himself from the stair banisters at the family home but, fortunately, the clothes line that he had chosen to hang himself with had broken under his weight. When he was seen by the psy-chiatrist, Alan had a red weal mark around his throat from the noose. He was staring at a fixed point on the floor. Every now and then he would groan deeply and whisper to himself. He kept repeating the words 'I'm for it . . . I'm for it now'. He would not make eye contact with the doctor and initially refused to answer questions.

His son said that the previous week Alan had stopped going to work as a bailiff after he found out that his wife was having an affair. He had watched her obsessively for 2 days not letting her out of his sight. Then a few days ago he had taken to his bed and lain there for hours and hours neither moving, speaking, eating nor drinking. He had talked about how everything was his fault and had at times appeared to be pleading with an unseen person to forgive him. He felt that he must have committed some unpardonable crime and that he should now be punished.

Armed with this information the psychiatrist talked to Mr Benson again. This time Mr Benson replied, albeit only briefly. He said that God was telling him that his wife had had to find another man because her husband had been so evil. He confessed that he had once had an affair himself many years before and that God had told him in the last week that He had punished Mr Benson with a slow-growing syphilis. His wife could be spared from the syphilis only if he killed himself. Once he was dead his wife could begin a clean life with another man.

What evidence is there that this is a psychotic illness?

There is evidence of severe psychomotor retarda-tion in the history where Mr Benson takes to his bed and lies there immobile. The retardation is so severe that Mr Benson sounds almost *stuporose*. More characteristic of psychosis still are the refer-ences to auditory hallucinations (pleading with an unseen person, God telling him about his guilt and punishment) and a secondary delusion of ill-health (syphilis). The patient's insight has been lost.

How high is the risk of this patient attempting suicide again?

The risk is very high indeed because the psychotic depression is still unchecked and Mr Benson's insight is lacking. The hallucinations he hears tell him that his wife will only be saved if he dies. Since he has just tried to hang himself he obviously finds it impossible to resist these ideas. Without adequate treatment another suicide attempt seems exceed-ingly likely. If Mr Benson were to attempt to leave the hospital it would be necessary to detain, assess and treat him under the relevant mental health legislation. Whilst he was in hospital he would need to be watched very carefully in case he tried to kill himself again on the ward.

Depression

- Depressive illness affects 10–18% of the adult population.
- Depressive illness in the community is largely untreated because patients generally do not seek medical help. Of those that do seek help only about 60% of those that see their family doctor are recognised as suffering from depression.
- Depressive illness is treatable — over 80% of cases can be resolved with adequate treatment.
- Treatment may include antidepressants (SSRIs, tricyclics, MIRA drugs or MAOIs), ECT (for severe or delusional depression) or psychotherapy for mild to moderate depression (particularly cognitive therapy).
- *Always* ask depressed patients about suicidal ideation and suicide plans.

Table 4.2 Clinical features of hypomania

Common
- Overactivity
- Insomnia
- Elation
- Distractibility
- Pressure of speech
- Flight of ideas
- Grandiosity
- Irritability
- Hostility
- Extravagance
- Disinhibition

Less common
- Delusions (grandiose)
- Increased alcohol intake
- Increased libido
- Auditory hallucinations

Uncommon
- Promiscuity
- Suicidal ideation

Mania

Elation, overactivity and insomnia are the classical features of mania (Table 4.2). Society has never tolerated the mentally ill very well, and perhaps because society finds manic patients particularly disruptive such patients are brought to the attention of the doctor relatively early. Cases are, therefore, relatively mild, and therefore termed *hypomania* rather than the more severe *mania*.

Mania has an earlier age of onset than depression (late adolescence/early adulthood) and more often has a familiy history. If one of a pair of identical twins suffers with bipolar affective disorder there is a 80% lifetime chance that the other twin will eventually suffer with the same illness, indicating a strong genetic component.

Mania can occur for the first time late in life, but it is then vital to exclude other physical causes such as hyperthyroidism or frontal lobe damage (perhaps due to a stroke).

Just as there is a persistent form of low mood termed *dysthymia* (not amounting to clinical depression), there is a mild form of alternating mood that corresponds to bipolar affective disorder. This persistent instability of mood involves many short lived episodes of depression and elation and is called *cyclothymia*, from the cycling nature of the mood. A few weeks' period of happiness and high productivity is replaced by a few weeks of low mood, low self-confidence and social withdrawal. Cyclothymia does not tend to come to medical attention because of its mild nature.

—| CASE HISTORY 3 |—————————

Elizabeth was a 27-year-old doctor who worked as a trainee in general practice. She had always been conscientious about her work and was keen to progress in her chosen career. Her practice colleagues had noticed a slight change in her over the previous days. She had seemed very cheerful and full of good humour, but one patient had complained to the receptionist that 'the young lady doctor was giggling when I told her about my infection'. Her colleagues assumed that perhaps Elizabeth was in high spirits because she was due to go on an all expenses paid conference at the weekend.

At the conference she made friends very freely and seemed very attached to a young doctor she had never met before. People in the audience around her were unnerved by the loudness of her laugh, however, and became embarrassed when she seemed to laugh rather too long after one speaker's presentation. Someone next to her whispered to her to be quiet. Elizabeth put out her tongue at this colleague and flounced out of the lecture room, slamming the door behind her.

That night she was sighted in the bar, drinking heavily and leering at a salesman who was running his hand up her thigh. They disappeared off to her room, but she was seen an hour later talking intimately to a different man in the coffee lounge. Her voice was loud and she was making very suggestive remarks that could be heard by the whole company.

The next day she was not to be seen in the conference room. Some delegates wondered what had become of her and made some cruel remarks about her.

The lecture by the local Professor of General Practice (a gentleman that Elizabeth was hoping to get an important research post with) was presenting a talk on 'Screening in General Practice'. His first slide had just been projected when a naked figure rushed from the side of the stage and hugged the eminent professor. There was a slight struggle whilst he tried to disentangle himself from Elizabeth. By this time she had removed the lapel mike from him and shouted into it: 'It's not screening in general practice you want, but screaming in general practice'. And so saying she began to scream into the microphone to the discomfort of the bewildered audience. A quick-thinking friend from Elizabeth's medical school days rushed onto the stage and, wrapping her in a coat, coaxed her offstage and took her to the hospital.

What features of mania did Elizabeth have?

The onset of the illness was during the week before the conference. Her patients noticed that she was less sympathetic to them, and even laughed at their troubles, suggesting a degree of disinhibition.

Her colleagues noticed that she was overly happy, but wrongly ascribed it to her forthcoming leave. At the conference itself Elizabeth becames progressively disinhibited: she talked loudly during presentations and later disrupted them by appearing naked. There is irritability (she storms out of the lecture theatre at one point) and some suggestion of promiscuity. An informant might be able to tell

you about Elizabeth's normal behaviour, but her approach to strangers sounds both unusual and potentially dangerous.

What risks does Elizabeth run?

Elizabeth's judgement is impaired because she is disinhibited. Her sexual approaches to strangers leave her vulnerable to abuse, assault, rape, unwanted pregnancy, venereal disease and HIV infection. We may assume that such approaches are not her normal behaviour.

Her physical safety is of primary importance, but there are other risks: her unusual behaviour prior to the conference may lead her to lose her professional standing in the practice (a patient might make a formal complaint about her manner or actions) and her bizarre behaviour at the conference could destroy her long-term career hopes. It is not unusual for people with affective disorders to lose their jobs or their marital partners long before a diagnosis of mental illness is made and treatment begun. Although in this vignette we are not told whether Elizabeth has grandiose ideas, it is common for manic people to feel wealthier than they in fact are. Manic individuals may make rash business decisions and overspend, for instance ordering a new car when they have no real means of paying, or running up huge credit card bills.

Psychiatrists, with their knowledge of mental illness, must act to protect such ill individuals from the consequences of their temporarily impaired judgement.

CASE HISTORY 4

Mr Unwin, 56, presented to casualty having assaulted a police officer and having caused a disturbance in a telephone box. The Registrar who was going to assess Mr Unwin heard him shouting and swearing loudly before opening the door of the assessment room. The Registrar introduced himself: 'Hello Mr Unwin? My name is Dr Brown . . . .'

Mr Unwin interrupted, 'Brown, green, blue what you going to do?' He paced the room, watched by the police constable who had escorted him to hospital. 'I've no time to waste, so make haste. I've got a hundred and one things to do, Dr

Blue. A hundred and one dalmations to give to the nations. The nation's going to the dogs. I have a plan to make a million before supper and I will not put up with the likes of you Dr Blue. Come on, come on, speak up!'

Mr Unwin himself spoke very rapidly indeed — so rapidly that it was hard to make out what he was saying. It was difficult for the doctor to get Mr Unwin to focus on any one issue because he was so easily distracted. At one point the sound of an aeroplane coming from outside made the patient pause. 'It's not easy,' he said. '500 people on that Jumbo. Rajah airways — and I'm responsible for everyone. I'm responsible for keeping the plane in the air. It's so difficult being God — having to keep touch with everyone and everything — you can't even go to sleep.'

It transpired that Mr Unwin had not slept for 3 days. He had not been drinking but had been found in a telephone box beating the receiver against the glass. He had become frustrated after the television station that he had been phoning hung up on him. 'If they'd let me on the television I could have stopped the war in Africa,' he said.

What features of this case suggest a manic illness?

Mr Unwin speaks rudely to the doctor (he is disinhibited); he speaks rapidly (pressure of speech) and displays flight of ideas. He uses rhyming associations. There is ample evidence of grandiosity (he believes he can stop the war in Africa and is deluded that he is God). He also displays some irritability.

What might the differential diagnosis be?

The illness sounds like an acute one, but if there was evidence of personality change over time you might need to exclude a frontal lobe tumour or an endocrine cause like hyperthyroidism. Head injuries and toxic states due to drugs or infection might present atypically in this way. In older men with hypertension and no past psychiatric history the possibility of a cerebral infarction should be excluded. The registrar should, therefore, be alert for any signs of an altered level of consciousness.

What lines of enquiry would help decide what the diagnosis was?

A past psychiatric history might reveal previous episodes of bipolar affective illness. An informant history would cover drug or alcohol use, physical ill health and recent personality change. A drug history might reveal whether lithium carbonate or antipsychotics have been used in the past and whether poor compliance with medication is a cause of relapse or not.

What management issues are important?

Mr Unwin probably has poor insight given that he has been acting on his grandiose ideas (phoning up television stations) and may not believe that he is ill. If he does not believe that he is ill he may well refuse to come into hospital. Mental health law may need to be used to compel him to be admitted. Once admitted he will need a full physical examination and relevant investigations. Treatment with antipsychotics may be necessary to control his manic symptoms in the short term and a mood stabilising drug started in the medium term. Suitable mood stabilisers might be lithium or carbamazepine. These would help prevent relapse or recurrence of the illness. Whilst in hospital, staff would need to protect Mr Unwin from the consequences of his illness (e.g. overspending behaviour and suicidal mood swings).

LEARNING POINTS

Mania

- Key symptoms of mania include overactivity and insomnia coexisting with either elation or irritability.
- Key signs of mania include restlessness, distractibility, irritability, pressure of speech or thought and disinhibition.
- Mania usually implies a bipolar affective illness and episodes of mania may be followed by episodes of depression.
- Despite elation and grandiose ideas the hypomanic patient may switch into a depressed or suicidal state.
- Doctors should endeavour to protect manic patients against the consequences of their poor judgement.

- Mania is much less common than depression.
- Mania has an earlier age of onset than depression.
- Acute treatment may include neuroleptics; prophylactic treatment may involve lithium or carbamazepine therapy.

Self-assessment

MCQs

1 Depression:
  a is more common in men than women
  b is usually treated by a psychiatrist
  c is often extremely difficult to diagnose
  d usually responds well to appropriate antidepressant therapy
  e is rare after the age of 70

2 Patients who are manic:
  a are best treated in their own home
  b may show irritability rather than elation
  c usually have their first episode of mania after the age of 40
  d may overspend
  e classically have paranoid delusions

3 Common symptoms of depression include:
  a nihilistic delusions
  b ideas of self-harm or suicide
  c disturbed sleep
  d derogatory auditory hallucinations
  e poor concentration

4 Biological (or somatic) features of depression include:
  a early morning wakening
  b mood worse in the mornings
  c psychomotor retardation
  d anorexia
  e loss of libido

Short-answer questions

1 What are the clinical features of mania and hypomania?
2 What kinds of delusions are associated with psychotic depression?
3 What is the prevalence of depression?
4 How can episodes of depression be treated and subsequently prevented from recurring?

MCQ answers

1 a = F, b = F, c = F, d = T, e = F
2 a = F, b = T, c = F, d = T, e = F
3 a = F, b = T, c = T, d = F, e = T
4 a = T, b = T, c = T, d = T, e = T

Explorations

Links with medicine

Many endocrine disorders are associated with affective illness, such as hypothyroidism and Cushing's disease. What other endocrine disorders are associated with affective illness? What could the links between physical illness and psychological symptoms be?

Links with obstetrics and gynaecology

What reasons could there be for an apparent excess of depression in females? What endocrine hypotheses exist for postnatal depression and premenstrual syndrome? What evidence is there for these hypotheses? Following childbirth what percentage of mothers experience the 'baby blues'? When are the 'baby blues' most likely to occur? How do the 'baby blues' differ from postnatal depression?

Links with surgery

Adverse life events are often associated with depression. Redundancy and bereavement are well-established risk factors for depression. Some surgical procedures such as mastectomy are associated with depression. Which other surgical procedures do you think would be particularly associated with later depression? What factors about such operations and diagnoses may provoke depression? What could services do to minimise suffering from depression after such operations?

Links with general practice

Ten per cent of all elderly people suffer with depression. Only about 5% of these cases of depression are treated. What can family doctors do to detect and treat these cases of depression? Loneliness, lack of satisfaction with life and bereavement are key risk factors for such depressive illness in the elderly. What can be done to prevent depressive illness?

Links with professional values/ethics

What percentage of junior and senior hospital doctors suffer with depression? In what way might depressed doctors underperform? How could you recognise depression in colleagues or yourself? What would you do about it?

■ Further reading and references ■

Texts

Brown G, Harris T 1978 The social origins of depression. Tavistock, London

Storr A 1990 Churchill's black dog and other phenomena of the human mind. Fontana, London

Papers

Chambers R 1993 Avoiding burnout in general practice. British Journal of General Practice 43: 442–3

Dinan T G 1994 Glucocorticoids and the genesis of depressive illness. British Journal of Psychiatry 164: 365–371

Green B H, Copeland J R M, Dewey M E et al. 1992 Risk factors for depression in old age. Acta Psychiatrica Scandinavica 86 (3): 213–7

Holden J M 1991 Postnatal depression: its nature, effects and identification using the Edinburgh Postnatal Depression scale. Birth 18(4): 211–21

Piccinelli M, Wilkinson G 1994 Outcome of depression in psychiatric settings. British Journal of Psychiatry 164: 297–304

Roy A 1985 Early parental separation and adult depression. Archives of General Psychiatry 37: 987–991

Sclare P, Creed F 1990 Life events and the onset of mania. British Journal of Psychiatry 156: 508–14

Weissman M M, Klerman G L 1977 Sex differences in the epidemiology of depression. Archives of General Psychiatry 34: 98–111

Affective disorders in literature

Lucas V (Sylvia Plath) 1964 The Bell Jar
Styron W 1991 Darkness Visible: A Memoir of Madness
Lehmann R 1981 The Weather in the Streets

■ Resources ■

Depression, Mania

Depressives Anonymous,
36 Chestnut Avenue,
Beverley,
North Humberside
HU17 9QU
Tel: 01482 860619
A national self-help association with local groups and open meetings.

Depressives Associated,
P O Box 1022,
London SE1 7QB

The Manic-Depression Fellowship,
8–10 High Street,
Kingston-upon-Thames,
Surrey KT1 1EY
Tel: 0181 974 6550
Fax: 0181 974 6600

Manic-Depression Fellowship (North-West)
Workspace,
23 New Mount Street,
Manchester M4 4DE
Tel: 0161 953 4105
The MD Fellowship educates the public about bipolar illness and publishes its own journal and newsletters. It runs self-help groups, open meetings and a pen-friend scheme. Its patron is Spike Milligan.

The Samaritans,
10 The Grove,
Slough SL1 1QP
Tel: 01345 909090
Fax: 01753 819004
E-mail service for suicidal and despairing: jo@-samaritans.org
Other e-mail: samaritans@cix.compulink.co.uk
The Samaritans has nearly 200 local branches manned by some 23 000 volunteers and takes nearly 2.5 million calls for help per year. It now offers an e-mail service whose electronic mail box is read daily.

MIND,
22 Harley Street,
London W1N 2ED.
Tel: 0171 637 0741

Postnatal depression

Association for Postnatal Illness,
25 Jerdan Place,

Hammersmith,
London SW6 1BE
Tel: 0171 386 0868

Meet-a-Mum Association,
14 Willis Road,
Croydon,
Surrey
Tel: 0181 665 0537
Fax: 0181 665 1972
Launched in 1979 by Esther Rantzen and *Woman* maga-
zine, MAMA aims to alleviate feelings of loneliness and
depression perinatally. It is essentially a charity which
coordinates a series of self-help groups.

National Childbirth Trust,
Alexandra House,
Oldham Terrace,
Acton,
London W3 6NH
Tel: 0181 992 8637

Bereavement

CRUSE — Bereavement Care,
Cruse House,
126 Sheen Road,

Richmond,
Surrey TW9 1UR
Tel: 0181 940 4818
Fax: 0181 940 7638
Cruse has 94 local branches and provides individual
and group counselling. Cruse has a 'Bereavement Line'
which provides a direct link to a counsellor: Mon-Fri
from 9.30 a.m. to 5.00 p.m. Tel: 0181 332 7227

Foundation for the Study of Infant Death,
Cot Death Research and Support,
35 Belgrave Square,
London SW1X 8QB
Tel: 0171 235 1721

For doctors

National Counselling Service for Sick Doctors,
1 Park Square West,
London NW1 4LJ
Tel: 0171 935 5982

Compassionate Friends (for bereaved parents),
53 North Street,
Bristol
BS3 1EN
Tel: 01272 539639

5

Suicide and assessing deliberate self-harm

There are about 1 500 000 suicide attempts every year in the European Community. Depression, schizophrenia, alcoholism and most other mental disorders greatly increase the risk of suicide. About 15% of people with affective disorders and 10% of people with schizophrenia eventually kill themselves. Careful assessment and management of psychiatric patients may help prevent some of these deaths.

Contents

Suicide

What is suicide?

Suicide is the deliberate taking of one's own life. Attempted suicides can be by a variety of means: self-poisoning (drug overdoses and the like), self-strangulation, failed attempts at hanging and so on. *Deliberate self-harm* is abnormal behaviour aimed at causing phsyical harm to the body but without clear intent to take life, such as repeated minor cutting of the wrists or forearms.

How common is suicide?

There are about 4500 recorded suicides in the United Kingdom every year. This works out as a recorded suicide every 2 hours. Suicide is about four times more common in men than in women, although there are more suicide attempts by women. Women are far more likely to choose drug overdoses as a method. In drug overdose there is a greater chance of intervention than in traditionally male means of attempting suicide such as hanging, gassing or firearms (see Fig. 5.1).

Risk factors for suicide

- Unemployed men are 2–3 times more likely to kill themselves.
- Certain occupations such as vets, doctors, dentists, pharmacists and farmers are at high risk.
- Single, widowed and divorced people are more likely to kill themselves than married or co-habiting people.
- About 10% of people with schizophrenia, 15% of alcoholics and 15% of people with affective disorders go on to kill themselves.
- Young people with conflicts about their sexuality.
- Drug misuse and homelessness.
- Terminal or disabling illness and chronic pain.
- Family history of suicidal behaviour.
- Loneliness and social isolation.

CASE HISTORY 1

Janet, 17, was brought to casualty by her sister. Janet had told her sister that she had taken a handful of her mother's antidepressant tablets to kill herself. The overdose had followed a row with her 18-year-old boyfriend, Darren.

She had secreted herself in her bedroom, drunk half a bottle of Pernod and swallowed the contents of a bottle containing her mother's imipramine tablets. She had written an angry letter to Darren, blaming him for ruining her life and causing her suicide. When she began to feel drowsy Janet felt scared and called down to her elder sister in the kitchen. The sister drove her to casualty with the empty bottle and the suicide note.

On admission Janet smelt of alcohol and was becoming unconscious.

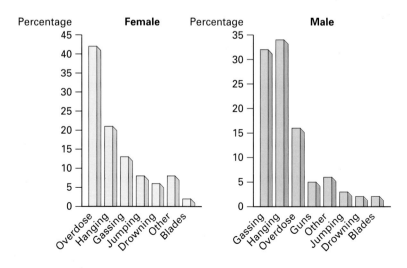

Fig. 5.1   Different methods of suicide in males and females.

What are the dangers associated with a toxic dose of tricyclic antidepressants?

Tricyclic antidepressant overdoses are difficult to manage. Drowsiness, coma, epileptic fits and cardiac problems may result. In addition to coma, anticholinergic activity may produce mydriasis, tachycardia and hallucinosis. Conduction abnormalities and myocardial depression are common. Doses above 2 or 3 g have a 20% mortality (because of hypotension and heart failure).

Initial management may include gastric lavage and repeated doses of activated charcoal. Correction of acidosis may prevent cardiac problems. Heart monitoring is essential in the initial stages and for some time afterwards. Ventricular arrhythmias and epileptic fits will require active intervention, say, with lignocaine or diazepam respectively.

On the day after the overdose what questions would a psychiatrist want to ask Janet?

The psychiatrist will be trying to assess whether Janet has a mental disorder and whether it is treatable. The psychiatrist will also want to try and assess whether there is an immediate risk of a further suicide attempt (and whether there is a risk of harm to others).

The psychiatrist will try to assess whether there is a treatable depressive illness by asking about depressive symptoms in the weeks leading up to the overdose (tearfulness, insomnia, anorexia, reduced libido and weight loss, for instance). Because alcohol was used in the overdose it would be important to assess whether Janet had an alcohol problem and questions about daily intake and symptoms of dependence would be warranted. In the mental state examination, questions used to elicit psychotic symptoms might determine whether there was a schizophrenic illness.

The psychiatrist will also try to assess how determined a suicide attempt this was — the type and number of pills taken is not a good guide to motivation, but things like precautions taken by the patient to avoid discovery suggest a certain determination to kill themselves.

A large number of overdose cases have an 'impulsive' quality to them. They sometimes follow a major family row, difficulties at school or work, or, as in Janet's case, a breakdown in a romance. Impulsive overdoses are made more likely by drinking alcohol because alcohol disinhibits the individual, making unwise decisions more likely. Overdoses can be the means of expressing anger or revenge (e.g. 'they'll miss me when I'm gone — they'll be sorry then') or of manipulating people — for instance forcing someone to their point of view (e.g. 'if you don't rehouse me today I'll kill myself').

Despite this unpleasant aspect, impulsive overdoses can be as fatal as any other kind. Paracetamol overdoses are notorious for their long-term effects on liver function. Days after the patient has regretted their paracetamol overdose, they may still succumb to hepatic failure. Overdoses are a common suicide method in women. Men opt for more violent means such as hanging, shooting or gassing. These more violent means are often more fatal and an 'impulsive' suicide attempt may be as fatal as a suicide attempt within the setting of longstanding mental illness.

CASE HISTORY 2

Adam was a farmer who lived by himself on a hill farm. He was aged 47 and had never married. He had no close relatives and, apart from a few drinking companions in the local pub, he had no friends. The village doctor had treated him for two depressive episodes when Adam was 30 and 35. In the past year he had had several setbacks. A large number of his flock of sheep had had to be destroyed after becoming infected. The bank had threatened to foreclose on his business loan. A government grant had failed to materialise and his hired help was suing him for negligence after a farming accident. The village doctor had diagnosed a depressive illness after Adam had come to the surgery complaining of sleeplessness. He had prescribed a course of antidepressants for Adam and arranged for a psychiatrist to visit him at home.

The next week the doctor was called to the farm by the village postman who was there to deliver a parcel. The doctor found Adam dead in the kitchen. He had shot himself in the head with his shotgun.

What factors suggested a high risk of suicide for Adam?

Adam lived alone, was single, male, had multiple financial and legal problems, had no support network and had a past psychiatric history. This case highlights the problem of working in remote areas where, perhaps, resources are few. In urban areas it might be easier to call in community psychiatric nurses and arrange day centre or day hospital attendance. Even so, it is unlikely that Adam would have attended day resources. Self-employed people find it difficult to take time off from their work. In this case the village doctor probably did everything he reasonably could. He correctly diagnosed the depressive illness. He correctly prescribed treatment and he arranged follow-up. Even so, the people who 'survive' suicide, i.e. the people who are left behind after someone else has killed themselves, are often left with a mixture of sadness, guilt and anger.

LEARNING POINTS

Suicide

- Males are particularly likely to choose violent and 'non-reversible' means of killing themselves.
- Loneliness, certain key occupations and psychiatric illness are all important risk factors for completed suicide.
- Always include questions about suicidal ideas and plans in your psychiatric assessment.
- Those left behind after a suicide need special attention for their own feelings of betrayal and sadness.
- Suicide is exceedingly rare in children, but becomes much more likely after adolescence and in young adulthood.

Deliberate self-harm

CASE HISTORY 3

Dawn was a regular attender at the accident and emergency department. She had been cutting her wrists and forearms regularly since the age of 13. She was now 18 and her arms were covered in scar tissue. One night she attended after a violent row with a young man at the hostel where she lived. She had been drinking vodka and was verbally abusive towards the doctor who saw her to stitch up a couple of lacerations on her wrist. She winced as he put the local anaesthetic injection into her skin.

'Why do you cut yourself if you're afraid of the pain?' He asked her.

'It doesn't hurt at the time,' she said. 'At the time nothing seems to matter. You just have to do it. Then you feel better. You feel better when you see the blood coming out.'

She denied any wish to kill herself, but did complain of poor sleep in the past week, so the accident and emergency doctor was careful to ask a psychiatrist to see Dawn before she was discharged from casualty.

Why did Dawn not feel any pain when she cut herself, but did feel pain when the anaesthetic injection was given?

Alcohol may have had some role in limiting the pain she felt at the time of the cutting, but in deliberate self-harm the patient is often dissociated into a state a bit like a trance. The awareness of the cutting and the awareness of the pain derived from it are split. Often the cutting provides a kind of relief after building tension over the previous hours or days. Dawn experiences the relief as she sees her own blood flow.

The relief from tension is a psychological reward for the cutting behaviour. Since the behaviour is associated with a reward, the behaviour is more likely to be repeated in the future. This explains why acts of deliberate self-harm are often repeated.

Deliberate self-harm is particularly common in younger patients, who are female and who have abnormal personality traits. Sexual abuse and poor relationship functioning are particularly associated.

LEARNING POINTS

Deliberate Self-harm

- Patients who self-harm often repeat the behaviour if it is associated with some reward.
- Deliberate self-harm patients may go on to kill themselves.

- Abnormal personalities are associated with deliberate self-harm behaviour, but like anybody else, abnormal personalities can suffer with treatable mental illness and so they must receive a careful assessment.
- Severity of inflicted harm is not a reliable guide as to the likelihood of completed suicide in the future.

■ **Self-assessment** ■

MCQs

1 Deliberate self-harm:
   a is associated with a history of childhood abuse
   b is often associated with alcohol abuse
   c patients never go on to kill themselves
   d may be re-inforced if associated with a psychological reward

2 Suicide is more likely:
   a in males than females
   b in the summer rather than the spring
   c in the elderly rather than the young
   d to be completed using violent means in males than females
   e among alcoholics than the general population
   f among dentists than the general public

Short answer questions

1 What risk factors would you consider in assessing a patient who has recently taken an overdose?
2 What public health or Government interventions aim to reduce the suicide rate?

3 What mental health problems might arise in the friend of someone who has killed themself?

MCQ answers

1 a = T,   b = T,   c = F,   d = T
2 a = T,   b = F,   c = T,   d = T,   e = T,   f = T

■ **Explorations** ■

1 There are about 4500 recorded suicides in the United Kingdom every year. Why is this likely to be an underestimate of the true number of suicides?
2 The ten occupations in Table 5.1 have the highest suicide rates in England and Wales. Using the Proportional Mortality Ratio (PMR) — the extent by which suicide is more or less frequent compared to the general population (a PMR of 100 would be the same as for the general public) — suggest which factors about these occupations make them more at risk.
3 Figure 5.2 shows the number of deaths from suicide

Table 5.1   Male suicides by occupation: the top ten

Occupation	PMR	Deaths
Vet	364	35
Pharmacist	217	51
Dental practitioner	204	38
Farmer	187	526
Medical practitioner	184	152
Therapist	181	10
Librarian	180	30
Typist, secretary	171	16
Social scientist	179	11
Chemist	169	70

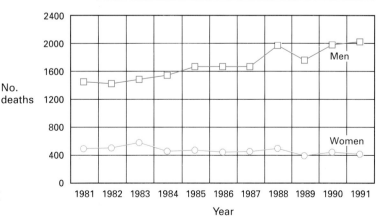

Fig. 5.2   Deaths from suicide and self-inflicted injury in young adults in the UK 1981–1991.

and self-inflicted injury in young men and young women (15–44) in the United Kingdom over the decade 1981–1991. What trends can you see? What would you predict from this trend? How could you investigate what actually happened in the years after 1991? What explanations might there be for the trend?

Further reading and references

CASEY P 1989 Personality disorder and suicidal intent. Acta Psychiatrica Scandinavica 79: 290–295

CHARLTON, et al. 1993 Suicide deaths in England and Wales. Population Trends, Edition 71

HAWTON K, CATALAN J 1987 Attempted suicide. A practical guide to its nature and management, 2nd edn. Oxford Medical Publications, Oxford

LONDON GAY TEENAGE PROJECT 1984 Something to tell you

KALTREIDER N B 1990 The impact of a medical student's suicide. Suicide and Life Threatening Behaviour 20: 195–205

KESSEL N 1965 Self-poisoning. British Medical Journal, ii, 1265–1270, 1336–1340

MURPHY G E, WETZEL R 1990 The lifetime risk of suicide in alcoholics. Archives of General Psychiatry 47: 383–392

RUNESON B, BESKOW J 1991 Reactions of suicide victims to interviews. Acta Psychiatrica Scandinavica 83: 169–73

MARZOK P, TIERNEY H, TARDIFF K et al. 1988 Increased risk of suicide in people with AIDS. Journal of the American Medical Association 259: 1333–1337

PAYKEL E S, PRUSOFF B A 1975 Suicide attempts and recent life events: a controlled comparison. Archives of General Psychiatry 32: 327–333

ROY A 1982 Suicide in chronic schizophrenia. British Journal of Psychiatry 141: 171–177

VAN DONGEN C J 1991 Experiences of family members after a suicide. Journal of Family Practice 33: 375–380

VARAH C 1965 The Samaritans. Constable, London

Suicide attempts and suicide in literature

BURGESS A. You've had your time

Resources

The Samaritans,
10 The Grove,
Slough SL1 1QP
Tel: (01753) 532713
Fax: (01753) 819004

Neuroses

Neuroses are a group of disorders with neurotic symptoms such as anxiety, panic or fear. Psychotic symptoms are usually absent. Neuroses are relatively common and for their sufferers are disabling. They are a major source of time lost from work.

Contents

Generalised anxiety disorder

Generalised anxiety disorder (anxiety neurosis) is an illness with two components: psychological and somatic. Psychological symptoms of anxiety include a fearful preoccupation with the future, but with a free-floating anxiety. In other words, the anxiety cannot be pinned down to any particular event or person. The somatic symptoms include tachycardia, palpitations, essential tremor, muscular tension, hypertension, dizziness, sweating, hyperventilation and epigastric discomfort. Anxiety is often a presenting symptom of depressive illness and it can be difficult to distinguish the two. Anxiety may also be the presenting symptom of physical disorders. Several physical causes of anxiety are listed in Table 6.1.

Panic disorder

In panic disorder the anxiety is felt in separate recurrent bouts (panic attacks). Somatic symptoms of palpitations and dizziness may predominate and the sufferer may feel that they are about to die. Depersonalisation and derealisation may accompany the attack. The sufferer tends to avoid the places where such attacks have occurred in the past. A series of panic attacks may precipitate agoraphobia. Sometimes sufferers overcome their fear by misusing alcohol (Dutch courage).

Table 6.1 Some physical causes of anxiety

Metabolic disorders
e.g. hypoglycaemia

CNS disorders
e.g. temporal lobe epilepsy

Endocrine disorders
e.g. hyperthyroidism,
    Addison's disease

External causes
- alcohol withdrawal
- benzodiazepine and other drug withdrawal
- theophylline and aminophylline
- caffeine
- experimental infusion of sodium lactate
- some bronchodilators, e.g. salbutamol
- other sympathomimetic drugs

It is important to exclude organic causes for anxiety and panic disorders. Thyrotoxicosis often presents with anxiety and mitral valve prolapse and cardiac arrhythmias are associated with panic attacks.

Phobias

A phobia is an excessive and somewhat irrational fear of some object or situation which is usually so disturbing that it leads to avoidance of that object or situation (avoidance behaviour). Avoiding the feared thing only makes further contact with it more anxiety provoking. Psychological treatment is, therefore, based on two principles: reducing the anxiety associated with the feared object and practising exposure to the feared object or situation.

About 8% of the general public have some kind of phobia.

Agoraphobia

Agoraphobia is literally a fear of the market place, but covers a fear of crowds, fear or travelling on public transport, an avoidance of social situations and a marked tendency to stay at home, rarely, if ever, venturing outside. Often panic attacks in shops and crowds may herald the avoidance behaviour of agoraphobia. Three-quarters of sufferers are women.

Specific phobias

Most people have fears of things like the dark or spiders or mice, but rarely do they dominate our existence. When the fears become preoccupying and the individual takes special steps to avoid the feared thing (like asking a neighbour to read through all magazines first to ensure that there are no pictures of spiders), then a minor fear of some particular thing becomes a specific phobia. Only about one in ten sufferers is male. Table 6.2 shows some specific phobias.

Social phobias

These involve the fear of meeting people or the fear of behaving in an out of the ordinary way in company. Whereas the agoraphobic is frightened of people in the mass, the social phobic is also often afraid

Table 6.2   Some specific phobias

- Birds
- Spiders
- Dogs
- Cats
- Mice and rats
- Moths
- Wasps
- Thunder
- Heights
- Darkness
- Flying
- Lifts
- Closed spaces
- Dentistry
- Doctors

of one-to-one interactions with others. Alcohol or benzodiazepines are often abused to reduce antici-patory anxiety ahead of the event. The anticipation causes anxiety which impairs performance in the feared situation leading to reduced confidence and more anxiety before the next meeting and so on.

Obsessive-compulsive disorder (OCD)

Obsessional ideas are repeated thoughts that come into a person's mind and which have some undesir-able quality to that person. The ideas may be non-sensical, violent or obscene. The sufferer often tries to resist dwelling on the ideas but to little avail. The ideas may be distressing, such as ideas about harming a baby in a new mother or swearing in a priest.

Obsessional ideas are sometimes called *intrusive thoughts*. Patients may describe them as being like a conversation in their head. The key points to distin-guish these *intrusive thoughts* from hallucinatory voices are that they:

- lack the real quality of a voice
- are experienced inside the sufferer's head (i.e. not experienced as external)
- are recognised as a product of the sufferer's own mind.

Neither are the intrusive thoughts delusional. Although the thoughts are sometimes incorrect, they can usually be challenged or the patient will volunteer how absurd the thoughts are. Nonethe-less, patients are tormented by them all the same.

Compulsive acts or rituals may be performed to reduce the anxiety associated with obsessional thoughts. For example, the person who continually fears contamination may wash and re-wash their hands many times a day. The compulsions, there-fore, are thought to ward off some undesirable event.

Performance of these rituals may interfere with everyday life. A patient who repeatedly spends 2 hours cleaning their hands after a toilet break at work may lose their job.

There is an overlap with depressive illness (since depressive illness may have obsessional features) and with obsessional personality. Obsessional per-sonalities are essentially meticulous and perfect-ionistic workers who, if given a deadline, will work to it, but who may expend great effort in getting things just right. Their attention to detail may infu-riate those around them.

Dissociation disorders

Imagine the mind has many layers of awareness. In clear consciousness we are aware of our surround-ings and our inner thoughts at all levels. A thought which occurs at one level is apparent throughout the system. The sensation of hunger at one level is accompanied by fantasies of food and plans of how to get that food at other levels. At other levels of the mind memories of past meals and events might be triggered too. Somehow the thoughts, memories and sensations on all these levels are integrated.

In dissociation disorders we might imagine that somehow the layers are not integrating properly so that there are discrepancies or dissociations between thought activity at different levels. Some people speak of a 'splitting of the stream of consciousness'. An example of this dissociation might be that some memories are seemingly unavailable to the con-scious individual. Hypnotic or trance-like states, and depersonalisation states, are other examples.

When something extremely unpleasant happens, dissociation may be a way of coping. Children who are being abused often feel as if the abuse is not hap-pening to them but to somebody else. They feel removed from it all. When the abuse is not happen-ing it may be difficult for them to access the memo-ries and feelings they had whilst they were being abused. Sometimes these split-off memories may only be acknowledged by the abused individual years later. The information about the unpleasant event is not lost but is stored at some relatively inaccessible level to protect the sufferer from hurt. A further example of dissociation is the phenomenon in battle where a soldier running across a battlefield is shot at but continues running oblivious of the bullet that has entered him. Only when he returns to safety can he begin to feel the pain and acknowledge the wound he has sustained.

The lack of integration caused by dissociation may produce a number of related disorders.

Sigmund Freud described a variety of cases, then diagnosed as hysteria, but which now attract the diagnosis of *dissociative conversion disorders.* An example might be a young patient who has no physical abnormality but who is adamant that they are unable to walk. The patient may undergo many diagnostic tests, but no abnormality is found. Other patients may present with atypical pains that defy our knowledge of human anatomy, or a sudden inability to talk (*aphonia*). The information about the unpleasant event is not lost, but is stored at some relatively inaccessible level to protect the sufferer from hurt. *Catharsis*, an emotional return to the original traumatic event via psychotherapy, hypnosis or drug abreaction (provoked by intravenous diazepam, say), may release the patient from their symptom. Often the symptoms have some symbolic meaning, so that a child who is frightened to speak out against the abuser may develop aphonia, i.e. the trauma is 'converted', hence the term *conversion disorder.*

Other dissociative disorders include dissociative amnesia (where important recent events are not recollected but there is no organic cause). The amnesia usually revolves around recent bereavement or traumatic accidents and is selective. Closely related to dissociative amnesia are dissociative fugues (wandering away from home coupled with amnesia and sometimes the assumption of a new identity) and dissociative stupor (psychomotor retardation in the absence of a history of depression, or loss of consciousness, often following some adverse event).

Somatisation disorder

Not all patients have the ability to formulate psychological distress in psychological or emotional terms. They may present their inner conflicts and distress as physical symptoms. At a basic level this may be 'a way in' to discussing their problems with their doctor, but at another level the patient may be quite unable to accept a psychological basis for their illness at all.

In somatisation disorder a patient may take their somatic symptoms from doctor to doctor in a vain attempt to find some test, investigation or cure that has not been offered elsewhere. Many negative investigations and therapies may have been tried by past doctors to no avail. Symptoms may involve any bodily system and include gastric pain, belching, vomiting, nausea, itching, burning, tingling and numbness amongst others.

Somatisers place doctors in a real dilemma. There is a temptation to pursue countless costly investigations to get a diagnosis, based on the knowledge that rare syndromes can sometimes present in such unorthodox ways. There is also a temptation to do nothing and wash one's hands of such difficult patients. Usually there is a deal of anxiety about when to stop physical investigations and begin psychological therapies. Patients usually are depressed and anxious themselves and specific antidepressant therapy may be warranted.

Confronting somatisers with 'the truth' is rarely helpful. They have usually received multiple reassurances that there is no physical explanation for their symptoms and resent the implication that they are not telling the truth. Attempting to help the patient make a link between the development and fluctuation of symptoms and life events and circumstances may produce results. However, the patient must 'own' the link themselves. It is no good for the doctor to present the entire theory out of the blue: it will not be accepted.

Psychiatric disorders occur in about 15% of general medical out-patients and in almost one-third of medical out-patients there is some degree of somatisation.

Adjustment disorders

When something unpleasant happens to someone — like a car accident, a bereavement or bad news about a physical illness — it takes time to adapt to this event. The individual will initially feel numb and may deny the situation before accepting that what has happened has happened, and become emotionally distressed. The distress usually affects the individual's ability to carry on their social and occupational roles. For a short time the individual may be unable to face work or friends. Ultimately, the individual may come to terms with what has happened and may form some means of coping with their changed life.

The time used to turn life round after an adverse life event can be referred to as a period of adjustment and the condition itself an *adjustment disorder*. The onset of the disorder is within a month of the event and the duration of symptoms is usually less than 6 months. If the disorder persists the diagnosis may be that of a depression.

Post-traumatic stress disorder

After severe life-threatening accidents or traumas, victims may suffer with a post-traumatic stress disorder (PTSD). PTSD is common in soldiers and it has been described in various wars. During the First World War it was known as 'shell shock'. Symptoms of PTSD include episodes of reliving the trauma. Reliving may occur in flashback sequences during the daytime or as *vivid recurrent dreams* during sleep. Other symptoms include hyperarousal, insomnia, social withdrawal, numbness, fear and avoidance of cues that trigger memories of the event. Reliving the trauma may be associated with anxiety, fear and aggression.

Depression may coexist with this disorder. Patients may also self-medicate with alcohol, and substance abuse problems are often associated with the disorder.

Antidepressant therapy may be helpful. Counselling as a matter of course is often offered to victims of disasters and those who witness them (e.g. stadium fires, crowd disasters), although there is no evidence for its efficacy.

CASE HISTORY 1

Alex would not shake hands when he came in to see the doctor. He looked at the two chairs in the doctor's room and chose the one that he thought looked least dirty. He perched on the very edge of the seat and folded his hands.

Alex told his doctor that he was sleeping badly

and that his degree work at the University was suffering. When the doctor asked about his sleep, Alex told him that he would lie awake worrying whether he had switched off all the lights or pulled out all the electric plugs in the living room or locked all the doors. He would get up to check not once, not twice, but at least 10 times. If he did not get up to check these things he was overwhelmed with anxiety until he did so. In addition, he was washing his hands up to 20 times a day to rid himself of germs. Whenever he went out of the house he always had to shower on his return and put on clean clothes.

He had always been a neat person and a meticulous worker. All his essays at University were done on a word-processor and laced with detailed references. However, in the last 2 months he had fallen behind on the deadlines for his essays because he had been checking and rechecking every sentence for mistakes. He was troubled by thoughts that he had become contaminated by other people. He had stopped seeing his girlfriend because he could not bear her to touch him lest she give him germs. He knew that the idea was illogical, but he could not stop thinking about contamination.

Is Alex suffering with a neurotic or a psychotic illness?

This is a very disabling illness — his relationships and work are being impaired. Despite this there are no psychotic symptoms. The thoughts of contamination coming into his head are not delusional (he knows that they are irrational) and the thoughts are clearly 'owned' by him (therefore ruling out thought insertion). These are examples of intrusive thoughts. Since there are no psychotic symptoms this disorder is more typical of a so-called neurotic illness.

What is the most likely diagnosis?

The intrusive thoughts and associated anxiety are typical of obsessional thought. The repeated checking behaviour which Alex does to reduce his anxiety is an example of compulsive behaviour. Alex feels compelled to check the light switches and plugs or else he is tormented by anxiety. Similarly, his obsessional fear about contamination is the basis for his compulsive handwashing. The most likely diagnosis is obsessive-compulsive disorder. Careful questioning would be justified to exclude a delusional basis for the obsessions, e.g. that extraterrestrials were deliberately conspiring to cover him with alien spores. Schizophrenia can sometimes present with some obsessive-compulsive behaviour. Nevertheless, as given above, the story is consistent with obsessive-compulsive disorder, not schizophrenia.

What treatments can be offered?

Some antidepressants with serotonergic activity are used to treat obsessive-compulsive disorder, namely fluoxetine and clomipramine. Either of these drugs may produce an improvement within a few weeks.

Psychological treatments include *thought stopping*, *response prevention* and *systematic desensitisation*. Thought stopping involves the patient voluntarily trying to distract him/herself from obsessional ruminations by, say, flicking a rubber band on the wrist. Response prevention may be carried out by a co-therapist attempting to prevent the patient from responding to obsessional impulses, for example, by stopping Alex from washing his hands and helping him seek alternative ways to reduce his anxiety. For fears of contamination the therapist may 'model' more adaptive behaviour, e.g. exposing him/herself and the patient to a graded hierarchy of increasingly dirty objects, working from dirty pullovers to dirty dishcloths and ultimately handling the contents of a waste basket. The patient follows the therapist's lead and models their behaviour on the therapist because the therapist handles the objects first.

─┤ CASE HISTORY 2 ├──────────

Elaine, 60, was a passenger in a car in a road traffic accident. She sustained a broken pelvis and spent some months in hospital. When she was discharged Elaine could not face travelling in a car again.

She went to her family doctor complaining of poor sleep with early morning wakening. She was also troubled with recurrent nightmares about the crash. During her waking hours she was haunted by sudden visual images of the accident coming

into her mind. 'It's as if it's all happening again,' she said. 'I'm there in the car again. I can see the other car coming towards us. I can hear the crashing metal. I can't get the smell of petrol out of my mind.' Anything on the television to do with cars brings the unwanted pictures and sensations back into her mind. Since television programmes and advertisements repeatedly feature cars, Elaine has stopped watching television altogether.

What additional features of Elaine's history would you want to know about?

A full history and examination would be essential in any psychiatric assessment, but her past psychiatric history and premorbid history are of special relevance. Does Elaine have a history of recurrent depressions or is this her first psychiatric presentation?

Her premorbid personality will give an indication of how well we can expect Elaine to be when she is well again. We also need to know about any other biological features of depression, suicidal ideation and any related alcohol abuse.

What are the main differential diagnoses?

The recurrent nightmares and daytime intrusive visual imagery (almost like being back in the accident) are fairly typical of post-traumatic stress disorder. Poor sleep is suggestive of a depressive illness, however, and a full history from Elaine and an informant would help us in our diagnosis.

How could Elaine be treated?

Antidepressants can be helpful in treating the depressive component of the disorder. Elaine's avoidance of certain stimuli (cars and television) could be reduced by using behavioural techniques, for instance by a desensitisation programme to cars.

─┤ CASE HISTORY 3 ├──────────

Olivia, 42, had been married for 22 years and had two teenage daughters. According to Olivia, the family is a very close one.

One day whilst shopping in town Olivia had a panic attack. She described it as 'being like a wave of anxiety that rolled my breath away. I stood there in the street shaking and staring.' She managed to get to a public telephone and called her husband at work. He came to pick her up and took her home.

Ever since then Olivia has been unable to leave the house alone. If her husband or one of her daughters accompanies her she can walk to the corner supermarket to buy small items of food. Even accompanied by other people she cannot face the weekly shopping trip to the hypermarket or venture into town. Unless her old friends call and see her she does not see anybody but her immediate family.

Her husband's career is a demanding one, but is beginning to pay dividends. He is being asked to head overseas sales trips on the company's behalf. He is very worried that Olivia's problem will mean he has to stay at home with her and he does not wish to lose his job.

In desperation, her husband asked the family doctor to make a home visit to see Olivia. When the doctor arrived he found Olivia tearful and guilty about the 'burden' she 'imposes on the family'. Even so she is adamant that she will never be able to go out alone again.

What are the likely diagnoses?

The low mood that Olivia displays could be a result of a depressive illness. The episode of illness begins with what sounds like a panic attack in the town centre. The attack seems to have been so frightening that Olivia has become sensitised to the place where she had the attack. She avoids similar places in case another attack is triggered. She has been conditioned to certain stimuli. The avoidance and fear of places like shopping centres is an example of agoraphobia. Whether the agoraphobia is part of the depression or vice versa is not known yet.

Panic attacks are sometimes caused by physical disorders such as thyrotoxicosis, epilepsy or mitral valve prolapse. These would need to be excluded.

What is the interaction between the illness and the family?

The illness requires not only the adaptation of the individual but the family as well. Everybody in the family has to adapt their lifestyle to help Olivia. This in itself provides some 'reward' for Olivia's behaviour and helps maintain the illness. Olivia would not consciously admit to using her illness to control the family. Nevertheless, this is the effect of the illness. At one level Olivia may be very worried about her husband's job and may ultimately perceive his success and trips abroad as a threat. Exploring the state of the marriage and the family dynamics would be important in helping the patient and her family. Sometimes illness is a form of communication. It may also be difficult for Olivia to say outright that she does not want her husband to travel abroad, or conversely she might know that he would not listen to such a message. He does though take account of her illness behaviour. However, 'blaming' Olivia for the illness will not help matters and any therapeutic initiative with the family must be carefully negotiated.

LEARNING POINTS

Neuroses

- Some neurotic disorders are relatively common: 14% of people suffer with a phobia, 2% from obsessive-compulsive disorder and 1.5% from panic disorder at some point in their lives.
- Neurotic disorders tend to be more common in women.
- Generalised anxiety disorders may be associated with depressive symptoms and self-medication with alcohol and other substances.
- Some psychotropic drugs can be useful in treatment, e.g. fluoxetine for obsessive–compulsive disorder and antidepressants where depressive symptoms co-exist with anxiety.
- Treatable physical causes of neurotic symptoms must be excluded initially, e.g. hyperthyroidism.
- Psychological treatments are particularly useful for neurotic disorders, e.g. desensitisation programmes for phobias and anxiety management groups for generalised anxiety or panic disorders.

Self-assessment

MCQs

1 Features of post-traumatic stress disorder include:
   a recurrent visual imagery

b recurrent nightmares
c auditory hallucinations
d feelings of fear or panic
e insomnia

2 Obsessive-compulsive disorder:
a usually involves intrusive ideas, images or impulses
b is much more common in women than men
c usually has its onset late in life
d often involves intrusive hallucinations
e may involve rituals that involve checking or cleanliness

3 Specific phobias:
a are usually accompanied by generalised anxiety
b usually manifest in middle age
c often involve avoidance behaviour
d may include a morbid fear of AIDS
e can be treated with desensitisation

Short answer questions

1 What is somatisation?
2 What treatments can be used for obsessive-compulsive disorder?
3 What investigations would you consider in a middle-aged woman presenting with anxiety?

Case vignette

Paul, a 34-year-old man, presented to his family doctor with feelings of panic associated with a dread of a forthcoming office party. He works as a porter in a large, local firm and is responsible for sorting and distributing the mail. He has only just got the job after years of unemployment. His boss is expecting all the workers to be at the party, but Paul has always avoided any social gathering with friends or family. In social situations he finds that he blushes and stammers and that people make fun of him. In the last few days he has begun drinking heavily which he finds calms his anxiety a bit. He smelled of alcohol to his doctor.

1 What problems does Paul describe?
2 What might the differential diagnosis be? What other information would you need to confirm a diagnosis?
3 What investigations might the doctor consider?
4 What management or treatment might the doctor suggest?

MCQ answers

1 a = T, b = T, c = F, d = T, e = T
2 a = T, b = F, c = F, d = F, e = T
3 a = T, b = F, c = T, d = T, e = T

Explorations

Links with physiology

What are the physical or somatic components of anxiety? How are the physical effects of anxiety mediated? What physiological systems are involved? How can this somatic component of anxiety be measured?

Links with pharmacology

Which neurotransmitter systems are responsible for producing somatic symptoms of anxiety? How can these effects be blocked?

Further reading and references

ANGST J, VOLLRATH M 1991 The natural history of anxiety disorder. Acta Psychiatrica Scandinavica 84: 446–452

CROFT-JEFFREYS C, WILKINSON G 1989 Estimated costs of neurotic disorder in UK general practice. Psychological Medicine 19: 549–558

DEANS H G, SKINNER P 1992 Doctors' views on anxiety management in general practice. Journal of the Royal Society of Medicine 85: 833–886

FREUD S, BREUER J 1895 Studies on Hysteria, vol. 1. Penguin Books, London

FREUD S 1915–1917 Introductory Lectures on Psychoanalysis, vol. 3. Penguin Books, London

GASK L, GOLDBERG D, PORTER R, CREED F 1989 The treatment of somatisation: evaluation of a training package with general practice trainees. Journal of Psychosomatic Research 33: 697–703

KAAYA S, GOLDBERG D, GASK L 1992 Management of somatic presentations of psychiatric illness in general medical settings. Evaluation of a new training course for general practitioners. Medical Education 26: 138–144

KIRMAYER I J, ROBBINS J M 1991 Three forms of somatization in primary care. Prevalence, co-occurrence and sociodemographic characteristics. Journal of Nervous and Mental Disorders 179: 647–655

PAWLIKOWSKA T, CHALDER T, HIRSCH S R, WALLACE P, WRIGHT D J M, WESSELY S C 1994 Population based study of fatigue and psychological distress. British Medical Journal 308: 763–6

VAN HEMERT A M et al 1993 Psychiatric disorders in relation to medical illness amongst patients of a general medical out-patient clinic. Psychological Medicine 23: 167–173

Neurotic symptoms in literature

DOSTOEVSKY F 1880 The Brothers Karamazov
DU MAURIER D 1938 Rebecca
FLAUBERT G 1874 The Temptation of St. Anthony
MURDOCH I 1985 The Good Apprentice
HODGSON-BURNETT F 1911 The Secret Garden
O'DOHERTY B 1992 The Strange case of Mademoiselle P

▄ Resources ▄▄▄▄▄▄▄▄▄

The Phobic Society,
4 Cheltenham Road,
Chorlton-cum-Hardy,
Manchester M21 1QN

Relaxation for Living,
168–170 Oatlands Drive,
Weybridge,
Surrey KT13 9ET

Trauma Aftercare Trust (TACT),
Buttfields,
The Farthings,
Withington,
Glos
GL54 4DF
Tel: 01242 890306

NO PANIC,
93 Brands Farm Way,
Randlay,
Telford,
Shropshire TF3 2JQ
Tel: 01952 590005; 01952 590545 (Helpline)

Phobic Action,
Claybury Grounds,
Manor Road,
Woodford Green,
Essex IG8 8PR
Tel: 0181 559 2551

7

Eating disorders

Eating disorders involve abnormal patterns of behaviour where people consistently eat too much or too little, and other behaviours such as bingeing and vomiting. Eating disorders are surprisingly common. There is a spectrum of eating disorders ranging from mildly abnormal attitudes about eating to severe anorexia nervosa.

Contents

Anorexia nervosa

The principal psychological problem is a morbid fear of fatness. In order to keep their body mass down the anorexic patient will diet excessively, combining this technique with strenuous exercise, the abuse of laxatives and diuretics and self-induced vomiting. Although the sufferer may be almost cachexic, he or she may see themselves as overweight. Sometimes such skeletal patients may draw self-portraits which are really caricatures of themselves showing themselves as obese.

One of the criteria used for the diagnosis of anorexia nervosa is a body mass 15% or more below the expected mass for a person of that age, sex and height (Fig. 7.1). Another criterion is amenorrhoea in women and loss of libido in men (secondary to reduced gonadotrophin levels because of self-starvation).

Young children and old people can be anorexia nervosa sufferers, but the preponderance of sufferers are teenagers. Ninety per cent or more of patients are women.

CASE HISTORY 1

Anna, 16, was brought to her family doctor by her worried mother. Her mother explained that her daughter was losing weight and looking increasingly frail and ill. With some difficulty she mentioned her fear that her daughter might have leukaemia or cancer. When the doctor asked about her daughter's appetite her mother said that Anna had 'gone off her food because she was too ill'.

From across the room the doctor could see how painfully thin Anna was, despite her having dressed in thick, baggy, woollen clothes. Although the weather outside was sunny, Anna's hands looked bluish and were cold to the touch. The doctor noted that there were abrasions on the knuckles of Anna's right hand.

How would you proceed with the interview?

There is a choice between continuing a conversation with the mother about Anna or interviewing Anna separately, possibly followed by the mother in

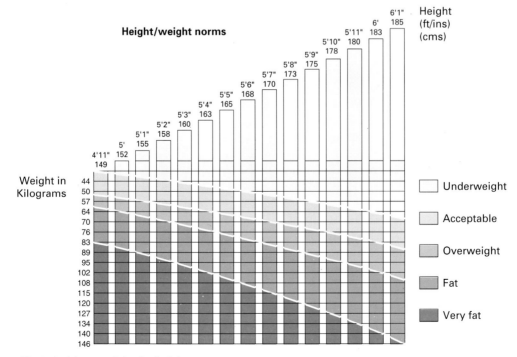

Fig. 7.1 Mean weights for heights.

turn on her own. Interviewing Anna on her own would allow you to assess her concerns and build a rapport with her. She is 16 and capable of answering for herself. Her cooperation will be essential whatever the diagnosis turns out to be.

Any medical illness must be excluded (Table 7.1), so the mother's fears will need to be explored. Questions to Anna might include 'What other symptoms you have noticed, Anna?' or 'What do you feel is the matter?'

If there is little history to suggest physical illness, questions should be asked about dieting behaviour and her feelings about her figure and appearance. More probing questions about her maximum ever weight and what her present weight is may encounter resistance, but should be asked.

What weight does Anna see as ideal (Fig. 7.2) Does she see herself as very thin? Have her periods

Table 7.1 The differential diagnosis of anorexia nervosa

Physical

- thyrotoxicosis
- malabsorption syndromes, e.g. coeliac disease
- malignant disease, e.g. leukaemia, oat cell carcinoma
- diabetes mellitus
- hypothalamo-pituitary
- tumours
- Crohn's disease

Psychological

- depression (with appetite loss)
- schizophrenia (with delusions involving food, e.g. that it is poisoned)
- bulimia nervosa
- abnormal eating attitudes

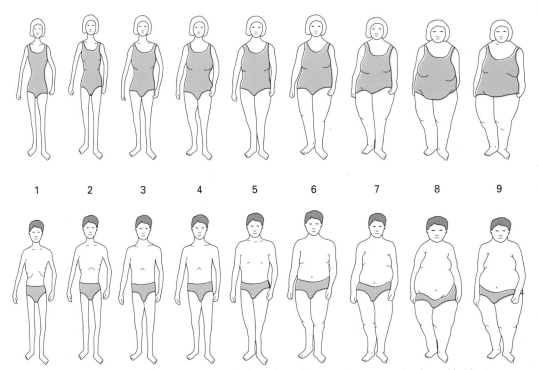

Fig. 7.2 Self-perceptions of attractiveness. Studies show that men (on average) selected body 4 as ideal for themselves and most attractive to women. Women (on average) thought they most looked like body 4 but wished they were thinner. Body three was the one they thought men would prefer.

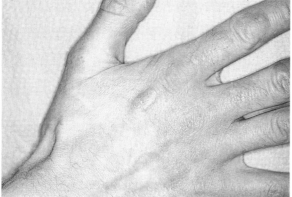

Fig. 7.3   Russell's sign of self-induced vomiting. Abrasions on the back of the hand are due to the skin rubbing against the teeth.

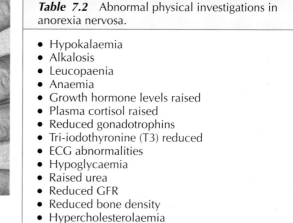

Table 7.2   Abnormal physical investigations in anorexia nervosa.

- Hypokalaemia
- Alkalosis
- Leucopaenia
- Anaemia
- Growth hormone levels raised
- Plasma cortisol raised
- Reduced gonadotrophins
- Tri-iodothyronine (T3) reduced
- ECG abnormalities
- Hypoglycaemia
- Raised urea
- Reduced GFR
- Reduced bone density
- Hypercholesterolaemia

stopped? How much food does she eat in a day? How often does she make herself sick? The abrasions on the dorsum of her hand suggest she makes herself sick by sticking her fingers down her throat. The abrasions arise because the skin rubs against the teeth (Fig. 7.3). Does she use laxatives or diuretics to reduce her weight? How much does she exercise? Can she concentrate on her schoolwork or is she constantly thinking about her weight?

This barrage of questions may generate vital information, but the experience is likely to feel unpleasant to Anna if she does have anorexia nervosa. Proceeding to an immediate physical examination may well humiliate her further, although such an examination does need to be done at some time. The doctor might make a mental note to do this at a subsequent visit, choosing to concentrate on gaining Anna's confidence on the first visit.

What physical features of anorexia nervosa might be found on physical examination?

The physical signs of anorexia nervosa are summarised in Figure 7.4.

What physical investigations might assist Anna's management?

Investigations would be used to seek the effects of long-term malnutrition and the severity of risk faced by the patient (Table 7.2). A full blood count will identify any anaemia and help exclude

any white cell dyscrasia. Urea and electrolyte screening will give a guide as to renal function and the possibility of hypokalaemia due to excessive vomiting. Thyroid function tests will exclude the differential diagnosis of thyrotoxicosis, but will also give a guide as to any secondary hypothyroidism associated with anorexia nervosa. A random glucose screen might help exclude diabetes mellitus. More specialised investigations such as growth hormone assays and an ECG might await any hospital referral.

CASE HISTORY 2

Mandy had been in hospital with anorexia nervosa for two weeks. Although she was 14 she looked much younger, and weighed only four and a half stone (28 kg). She had been admitted after fainting at boarding school. Since admission she had been put on to bed rest and kept in a private room. Visits by her family and phone calls to them were strictly regulated. Visits and phone calls were used as rewards by the nursing staff for eating her high-calorie diet (3000 kcal/day). Every Monday and Thursday Mandy was weighed to see if her weight was improving. If there was improvement then she was rewarded by greater freedom. In her first few days in hospital the nurses had noted that even though Mandy was eating her food, she was vomiting it down the sink unit in her room as soon as the nurse left the room with her empty tray. Nurses had also noticed that on the days she was weighed Mandy would try to drink as much water as she could just before she was weighed. Since noticing these things the nurses had watched Mandy very closely, which she did not like at all.

In her third week she had confided in a female occupational therapist that for a long time she had been receiving the unwanted sexual attentions of her form teacher. Staff acted to protect Mandy and to resolve family issues, as well as encouraging Mandy to gain weight. Three months after her weight returned to the average for her age, Mandy's periods re-started.

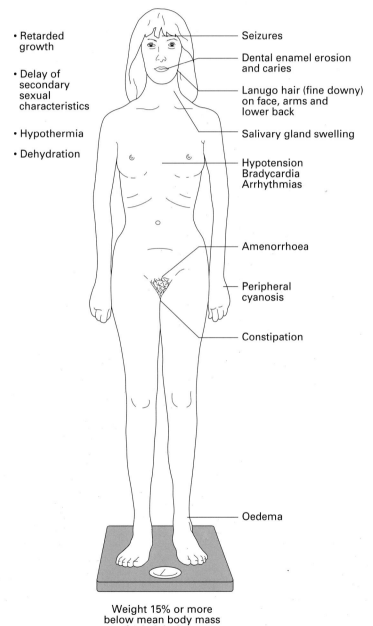

- Retarded growth
- Delay of secondary sexual characteristics
- Hypothermia
- Dehydration

Seizures

Dental enamel erosion and caries

Lanugo hair (fine downy) on face, arms and lower back

Salivary gland swelling

Hypotension
Bradycardia
Arrhythmias

Amenorrhoea

Peripheral cyanosis

Constipation

Oedema

Weight 15% or more below mean body mass for height / age

Fig. 7.4 Physical features of anorexia nervosa.

What made Mandy faint at school?

The metabolism of anorexic patients is mainly catabolic, and they are prone to hypoglycaemia. Cardiac arrhythmias and hypotension also predispose to syncope. School is also the place where her abusing teacher was, and the stress of this situation may also have been a contributing factor.

What are the aims of her hospital admission?

In severe anorexia nervosa the physical state of the patient may warrant admission for re-feeding and to correct any metabolic abnormalities. There is a substantial mortality associated with anorexia nervosa. Long-term follow-up studies show a mortality rate of 15–20% over 10–20 years (causes of death include frank starvation and oesophageal rupture). For this reason re-feeding is not the only aim of admission. Although some psychological factors can be caused or worsened by starvation (e.g. cognitive impairment, social withdrawal, irritability, depression and preoccupation with food), anorexic tendencies persist after re-feeding. After discharge from hospital relapse is, unfortunately, common. To prevent relapse other work needs to be done: educating the patient about the illness, about nutrition and the body's needs, and psychotherapeutic work with the patient and the family. Occasionally chlorpromazine or amitryptiline may be prescribed (both stimulate appetite and weight gain). Some new antidepressants like fluoxetine help with the preoccupation with food.

What role did the sexual abuse play in the genesis of Mandy's illness?

It has been estimated that up to 50% of anorexics have been sexually abused (set against a community prevalence of 20–30%). Some people see anorexia nervosa as the pubertal teenager's way of rejecting adult sexuality. Put together with a previous history of abuse, you can see why the sufferer might starve themselves to delay the onset of puberty and avoid the complications of adopting an adult shape.

Other people see anorexia nervosa as a 'battle for control' over the patient's body. In a world where the sufferer perceives himself or herself to be relatively helpless, it is sometimes a relief to at least be able to control their eating habits (although ultimately to their own detriment). The control itself is of paramount importance. This is why helping some anorexic patients can feel like a battle for control for their families and their doctors. The 'battle for control' model can fit in with the sexual abuse theory too, because in sexual abuse the victim often feels helplessly out of control and seeks any means of establishing some control over the outside world.

Although sexual abuse is an important factor in some cases, it must be remembered that abuse may not be present in others.

LEARNING POINTS

Anorexia nervosa

- Anorexia nervosa involves overvalued ideas about weight and shape — a 'morbid fear of fatness' and a preoccupation with food and its calorific value.
- Weight loss of 15% or more below norm for age/sex/height is a key diagnostic criterion.
- Ninety per cent of sufferers are female.
- Amenorrhoea in teenage women and low sex drive in boys are other key criteria.
- Anorexia nervosa is associated with multiple physical signs and metabolic complications.
- Physical causes of emaciation should be excluded (e.g. Crohn's or malabsorption syndromes).
- Patients may use a variety of covert means to keep their weight low (e.g. secret vomiting).
- Long-term mortality is high (15–20%).
- Gaining the patient's trust helps long-term compliance.
- High-calorie diets may be needed to reverse starvation.
- In-patient units may use behavioural management regimes (preventing vomiting and other means of reducing weight and drawing up a programme of weight goals and associated rewards).
- Individual and family therapy help prevent relapse.
- There is an association with child sexual abuse.
- Anorexia nervosa is more common in higher socio-economic classes (community prevalence 1% of women) and in higher educational settings (2–3% of women).

Bulimia nervosa

Bulimia nervosa differs from anorexia nervosa in three key respects:

- the body weight may be normal or excessive and periods may be present (although sometimes irregular)
- frequent binge eating
- more common than anorexia nervosa (2–3% of all women).

The sufferer is usually female and older than those with anorexia nervosa (presenting in their 20s). Although anorexics display a profound control over their eating behaviour, bulimics are characterised by their lack of control. Although concerned about their weight for most of the time, uncontrollable impulses may lead sufferers to binge on high-calorie foods. A typical binge might involve a tub of ice-cream and a packet of chocolate biscuits followed by half-a-loaf's worth of buttered toast. After such a binge the bulimic patient commonly feels extreme remorse and is thrown into despair. Self-induced vomiting may re-establish some self-esteem, but generally the self-esteem of bulimic patients is very low.

Clinical features

The clinical features of bulimia nervosa are summarised in Table 7.3. Parotid enlargement (Fig. 7.5) and dental erosion (Figs 7.6 & 7.7) are obvious features.

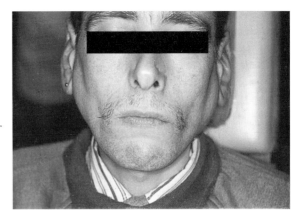

Fig. 7.5 Parotid enlargement.

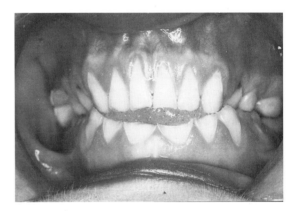

Fig. 7.6 Marked dental erosion produced by gastric acid during vomiting.

Table 7.3 Clinical features of bulimia nervosa
<ul><li>Past history of anorexia nervosa common (in about a third)</li><li>Frequent binge eating</li><li>Concern about weight and shape</li><li>Guilt and low self-esteem</li><li>Vomiting, laxative abuse and diuretic abuse, moderate exercise all used to try and reassert control</li><li>Irregular or absent menses</li><li>Dental decay (due to gastric acid)</li><li>Parotid gland enlargement</li><li>Calluses on the dorsum of the hand</li><li>Normal, high or low weight</li><li>Alkalosis, hypokalaemia</li><li>Electrolyte imbalance</li></ul>

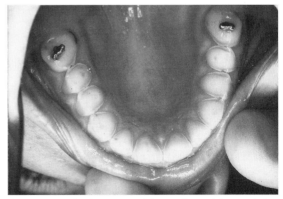

Fig. 7.7 Marked erosion of the surface of the teeth by acid to the extent that even the dental pulp has been exposed.

CASE HISTORY 3

Shortly after her wedding to Michael, Andrea attended her family doctor. She looked quite fit and well, but began by talking about how tired she was feeling and how unsympathetic her husband was. Picking up on her cues her doctor asked about the experience of being a newly wed. He went on to ask about the quality of their sexual relationship and it was at this point in the consultation that Andrea felt able to unburden herself.

Now aged 24, Andrea had been sexually active with several boyfriends in the past. This her family doctor already knew, but he was surprised to hear that every relationship had had the same pattern to it. At first Andrea had been head over heels in love with each new boyfriend and their sexual relationship had been marked by its intensity and freedom. Soon after the beginning of each relationship Andrea would feel an overwhelming guilt and an irresistible urge to stop seeing the boyfriend. This had led to a large number of very short, but very intense relationships, some of them little more than 'one night stands'.

Andrea had met her husband only 2 months before. Theirs was a whirlwind romance and the honeymoon had been graced by a closeness that Andrea had at first enjoyed, but now found oppressive.

To make matters worse she had begun doing something she had not done for many years. She had started raiding the fridge in the middle of the night and gorging herself on food which she had stocked there over the past few days. She would eat a family size trifle in a matter of seconds and follow it by a plate of salami and mayonnaise, then chocolate biscuits on which she had sprayed whipped cream. A few minutes after gorging herself she would go to the bathroom and stick her fingers down her throat to make herself sick. Full of guilt and despair she would return to her marital bed and lie awake thinking about what a bad and fat person she had become.

She had found that a hefty measure of sherry sometimes sent her off to sleep straight away and was enough to prevent her going downstairs to the fridge. Unfortunately Andrea had begun to see this as an occasional way of keeping bad feelings about herself at bay during the day. Every few days she bought a bottle of sherry and drank it steadily through the day, finishing it last thing at night.

What can the family doctor do to help?

The diagnosis of bulimia nervosa is a fairly clear one. There are repeated binges on highly calorific food, low self-esteem, feelings of fatness and the patient has a 'normal' appearance, like many bulimic patients (which is why the behaviour often goes undetected for many years).

The family doctor notices that there are echoes of this 'bingeing' behaviour in the rest of her life — there is a repeating 'bingeing' on men and alcohol. Like the food after a binge, the men are discarded once Andrea is racked by guilt. The family doctor might worry here about how Andrea's bulimic behaviour patterns could jeopardise her marriage.

The family doctor needs to collect more data about the extent of the bingeing behaviour and help the patient see a link between her feelings and behaviour and the events in her life. One way of raising these issues is to use self-treatment manuals. Sometimes doctors treating eating disorders ask their patients to complete a food diary for each day (Fig. 7.8). The diary logs food eaten, vomiting behaviour, events and feelings at various times through the day. Reading through the diary with the patient can help both doctor and patient see the pattern of behaviour – what things trigger bulimic behaviour? Such diaries can be used in a special kind of psychotherapy known as *cognitive-behavioural therapy*. Other forms of psychotherapy used to help can be individual dynamic psychotherapy and group therapy.

Some psychiatrists see such behaviour as resulting from disturbances in hypothalamic function. Since serotonin has been found to be important in the regulation of the hypothalamic appetite centre, the regular use of selective serotonin re-uptake inhibitors (SSRIs) has been found useful in reducing the frequency and severity of bulimic binges. An example would be fluoxetine 40–60 mg daily.

LEARNING POINTS

Bulimia nervosa

- Prevalence about 2% — presentations are mainly women in their 20s.

Day   Monday
Date   11/4/95

Time	Food Eaten and Drinks Consumed	Place	Binge	Vomiting	Events around eating	Feelings
8.15 am	1 grapefruit 1 orange black tea	Lounge			Watching breakfast TV	Anxious about day
10.15 am	16 choc biscuits sweet tea	Supermarket at Cafe	Binge		Tempted whilst shopping	Felt hungry
10.30 am		Supermarket at toilets		Vomit		Guilty Feel fat
Noon	Ate nothing Black coffee					Making up after binge
4.00 pm	Two Mars bars	Way home from shops	Binge			
4.10 pm		Home		Vomit		Felt sick
7.00 pm	Spaghetti bolognese Glass of wine	Dining room			Listening to Radio	Feel lonely, fat and unwanted
10.00 pm	half litre of choc ice cream, half a loaf, 2 bowls of cornflakes, 4 defrosted cream cakes, half bottle of wine	Bedroom floor	Binge			Feeling bloated and guilty
11.00 pm		Bathroom toilet		Vomit		Feel dreadful, can't sleep. Take sleeping tablet

Fig. 7.8 Example of a food diary kept by a bulimic patient.

- Weight may be normal, high or low.
- There is a loss of control over eating and sometimes over other behaviours such as alcohol or sex.
- Frequent binges of high calorie food a main characteristic.
- Associated with low self-esteem.
- Relatively few physical signs on examination.
- Patients may have a past history of anorexia nervosa or obesity.
- Psychological treatments include cognitive behavioural therapy, individual dynamic therapy and family therapy.
- Drug treatments include SSRIs and other antidepressants.

Obesity

Obesity is the commonest form of malnutrition in the developed world. Possibly as many as 30% of adults are more than 20% overweight. Extreme obesity is associated with excess mortality from a variety of causes including cardiovascular disease, diabetes mellitus, respiratory dysfunction and gallstones. Obesity is also associated with social, psychological and occupational difficulties. Obesity is seven to twelve times more common in low socioeconomic groups. Genetic factors seem to play a large part too, accounting for a significant proportion of the variance of the body mass index (Table 7.4).

Overweight people consistently underestimate their food intake and overestimate their energy expenditure by as much as 50%.

Obese people are often subject to low self-esteem and prejudice. Such prejudice and loneliness leads

Table 7.4 Differential diagnosis of obesity

Common causes
- excess calorie intake
- low physical activity

Rare causes
- endocrine causes (hypothyroidism, Cushing's disease)
- hypothalamic lesions
- insulinomas
- rare genetic causes, e.g. Prader-Willi syndrome

Table 7.5 Treatment initiatives in obesity

First-line
- calorie restriction
- exercise
- Weight Watchers or similar group

Second-line
- psychotherapy/cognitive-behavioural therapy
- total fasting (only with close medical supervision)
- fluoxetine
- amphetamines

Last resort
- gastric reduction surgery
- jejunoileal bypass

to further 'comfort eating' and a resultant worsening of the obesity. Intervention can interrupt this cycle, but up to now obesity problems form an insignificant part of the psychiatrist's workload (Table 7.5).

Health benefits can accrue from only a 10% reduction in weight. Diets, however, have their problems too. There is some evidence to show that weight instability (through alternating periods of dieting and overeating) may be more damaging than weight stability, even at an overweight level.

LEARNING POINTS

Obesity

- Excess weight increases morbidity and mortality from cardiovascular disease.
- Weight instability increases the relative risk of death over and above weight stability.
- Social, economic and genetic factors play their part in the aetiology of obesity.
- Overweight people underestimate their calorie intake and overestimate their energy expenditure.
- Health benefits may begin to accrue from modest weight loss (10%).
- Treatment options include low-calorie diets, moderate exercise programmes, self-help and commercial programmes, cognitive therapy, pharmacotherapy (e.g. fluoxetine or fenfluramine) for those more than 30% overweight, and possible surgery for people 100% or more overweight.

Self-assessment

MCQs

1 Clinical features of anorexia nervosa include:
- **a** loss of secondary sexual characteristics
- **b** a morbid desire for food
- **c** reduced growth hormone serum levels
- **d** leucopenia
- **e** raised serum levels of tri-iodothyronine

2 Anorexia nervosa:
- **a** involves intrusive delusional ideas about food
- **b** is best treated by psychoanalysis
- **c** can be diagnosed only when 25% of body mass is lost
- **d** affects less than 1/1000 teenage women
- **e** involves a dread of fatness which is an overvalued idea

3 Generally available treatments for bulimia nervosa include:
- **a** intensive psychoanalysis
- **b** family therapy
- **c** fluoxetine
- **d** cognitive behavioural therapy
- **e** risperidone

Short answer questions

1 List 10 physical complications of anorexia nervosa.
2 Explain the similarities and differences between anorexia nervosa and bulimia nervosa.

Essay

Describe the principles of the management of severe anorexia nervosa.

MCQ answers

1 a = F, b = F, c = F, d = T, e = F
2 a = F, b = F, c = F, d = F, e = T
3 a = F, b = T, c = T, d = T, e = F

Explorations

Links with physiology and biochemistry

What biochemical changes in metabolism are associ-ated with starvation? What calorific intakes are required for differing lifestyles? What psychological changes are associated with biochemical changes in starvation?

Links with epidemiology research

How would you design research to establish the prevalence of anorexia nervosa in a community? How would you design research to establish the outcome of a treatment for anorexia nervosa?

Links with community medicine/general practice

What self help groups and voluntary organisations exist for anorexia nervosa and bulimia nervosa sufferers? How can you assess the quality of the service they offer? What would the benefits and disadvantages be to clients of these services?

Further reading and references

BRUCH H 1978 The golden cage: the enigma of anorexia nervosa. Open Books, London

CRISP A H 1980 Anorexia nervosa: let me be. Academic Press, London

FAIRBURN C, COOPER P 1989 In: Cognitive behaviour therapy for psychiatric problems. A practical guide. Hawton K et al. (eds) Oxford Medical Publications, Oxford

HSU L K G 1990 Eating disorders. Guilford Press, New York

KING M B 1989 Eating disorders in a general practice population: prevalence, characteristics and follow-up at 12–18 months. Psychological Medicine, suppl. 14. Cambridge University Press, Cambridge

MANN A H, WAKELING A, WOOD K. et al. 1983 Screening for abnormal eating attitudes and psychiatric morbidity in an unselected population of 15-year-old schoolgirls. Psychological Medicine 13: 573–580.

PALMER R L 1989 Anorexia nervosa. A guide for sufferers and their families, 2nd edn. Penguin, London

RATHNER G, MESSNER K 1993 Detection of eating disorders in a small rural town: an epidemiological study. Psychological Medicine 23: 175–184

RUSSELL G F M 1979 Bulimia nervosa: an ominous variant of anorexia nervosa. Psychological Medicine 9: 429

RUSSELL G F M et al. 1987 An evaluation of family therapy in anorexia nervosa and bulimia nervosa. Archives of General Psychiatry 44: 1047

SHARP C W, Freeman C P L 1993 The medical complications of anorexia nervosa. British Journal of Psychiatry 162: 452–462

TREASURE J, SCHMIDT U, TROOP N et al. 1994 First step in managing bulimia nervosa: controlled trial of therapeutic manual. British Medical Journal 308: 686–689

Anorexia nervosa in literature

SHUTE J. Life-size
MACLEOD S. The Art of Starvation

Resources

Eating Disorders Association
Sackville Place,
44 Magdalen Street,
Norwich,
Norfolk NR3 1JU,
United Kingdom.
Tel: 01603 621414 (Mon–Fri 9–6.30 p.m.)
     01603 765050 (Youth helpline 4–6.30 p.m.)

Addiction

A wide variety of exogenous substances have addictive properties. Naturally occurring substances such as tobacco and cannabis have been used by man for thousands of years. Synthesised compounds such as alcohol, benzodiazepines, heroin and cocaine have become available in the last few centuries. For a substance to be addictive it must provide some psychological reward, e.g. relief of anxiety, and be capable of inducing dependence. Substance addicts often crave the substance when it is not available because of withdrawal effects.

Contents

Addiction, tolerance, dependence and withdrawal

Addiction is defined differently by different people. In this book addiction refers to a state of craving for a particular external substance which, for various reasons, the addict feels he or she needs and cannot do without. Addicts often act in ways that damage themselves or others in order to get and use the desired substance. Repeated exposure to the same dose may result in a diminishing response. This is known as *tolerance*, where the addict feels that they need to up the dose to achieve the same effect as before. *Dependence* can be physical or psychological. Abusers of alcohol may drink in order to cope with stressful situations. Without alcohol they may feel unable to cope. Physical dependence implies that there are physical symptoms when the drug is withdrawn, i.e. a *withdrawal syndrome*.

An example of a *dependency cycle* is given in Figure 8.1. In this cycle the use of an anxiolytic, e.g. a benzodiazepine, is prompted by anxiety, but once the benzodiazepine is metabolised the anxiety returns prompting reuse. Since benzodiazepines are associated with tolerance and withdrawal effects, there is a drive to take higher and higher doses more often to reduce anxiety. The faster the cycle spins the greater the risk of addiction. Short-lasting drugs spin the cycle quicker than long-lasting drugs so that benzodiazepines with short half-lives are more addictive than those with long half-lives. Table 8.1 gives the half-lives of various benzodiazepines.

Long-term benzodiazepine use is associated with a notorious withdrawal syndrome which includes rebound anxiety, rebound insomnia and convulsions. Some of the symptoms are given in Table 8.2.

Clinical features of addiction

These include:

- tolerance

Table 8.1   The half-lives of four benzodiazepines

Drug	$t_{\frac{1}{2}}(b)$ (hours)	Volume of distribution (l/kg)	% bound to plasma proteins
Chlordiazepoxide	6–28	0.3–0.6	95
Diazepam	20–40	1–2	98
Temazepam	8–16	1.3–1.6	97
Nitrazepam	18–31	1.5–2.8	87

Table 8.2   Some withdrawal symptoms associated with long-term benzodiazepine use

- Excitability
- Depersonalisation
- Poor concentration
- Illusions
- Hallucinations
- Obsessions
- Phobic behaviour
- Panic
- Rebound anxiety
- Depression
- Craving
- Rebound insomnia
- Vivid dreams
- Pain
- Paraesthesia
- Stiffness
- Formication
- Weakness
- Tremor
- Muscle twitches and fasciculation
- Ataxia
- Blurred vision
- Tinnitus
- Dysarthria
- Hyperacusis
- Convulsions
- Temporal lobe fits
- Nausea
- Vomiting
- Diarrhoea
- Constipation
- Dry mouth
- Metallic taste
- Dysphagia
- Flushing, sweating
- Palpitations
- Hyperventilation
- Thirst
- Frequency
- Polyuria
- Incontinence
- Menorrhagia
- Mammary pain
- Loss of libido
- Impotence
- Skin rash
- Stuffy nose

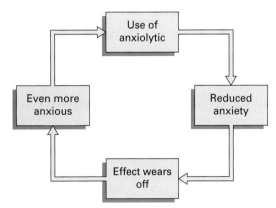

Fig. 8.1   The dependency cycle produced by anxiolytics.

- persistent desire for the substance
- unsuccessful attempts to cut down or stop using
- a great deal of time, effort or risk expended in obtaining the substance
- difficulty fulfilling social obligations at work, college or home
- persistent use despite awareness of adverse effects of drug on health or well-being of self or others
- withdrawal symptoms
- substance taken to avoid withdrawal symptoms.

The epidemiology of addiction

It is difficult to get true figures for the prevalence and incidence of substance abuse. For alcohol consumption epidemiologists look at Government revenue statistics on alcohol sales tax, population surveys and sometimes use indirect, but correlated, data such as deaths from liver cirrhosis. Certain occupational groups are at high risk of alcoholism: publicans, bar tenders, businessmen, service personnel, doctors and lawyers. In general hospitals 20–30% of all male admissions and 5–10% of all female admissions are probably heavy drinkers. At least 5% of all men and about 2% of all women in the UK have a drinking problem.

Statistics for illicit drug consumption are more difficult to obtain since there is no legal duty on illicit drugs. Information only arises, therefore, when addicts come into contact with official departments, e.g. doctors in the UK must notify the Home Office of addicts of certain controlled substances. Most notifications concern opiate addicts. Substance abuse is generally more common in men than women. Other information comes from criminal statistics, drug seizures, offences against drug laws and self-report surveys. Regular drug use in inner city schools may be as high as 20% of 16 year olds and is rising. In 1991 in the USA at least 40% of males arrested for burglary and assault tested positive for some drug. Between 9 and 64% of these drug users were using cocaine. Addicts indulge in a variety of crimes to get the money they need to fuel their addiction. Some of these may put them at particular risk of HIV infection, e.g. prostitution.

Psychiatric consequences of alcohol abuse

There are consequences for the individual, their family and society.

Individual consequences

The features of the dependence syndrome mean that the individual underperforms at work, socially and in the family. These factors, and disinhibition together with impotence, may threaten the alcoholic's sexual partnerships. Craving alcohol and its dominance of the waking hours may mean other activities are excluded and the alcoholic's life begins to revolve only around alcohol.

A *withdrawal syndrome* begins 8–24 hours after a persistently heavy drinker stops drinking. Withdrawal symptoms include: anxiety, convulsions, tremor, sweating, insomnia and loss of appetite. Withdrawal signs include: pupillary dilatation, tachycardia and raised blood pressure.

Delirium tremens is an acute confusional state which may occur 24–96 hours after stopping drinking. Symptoms include marked tremor, restlessness, disorientation, illusions and hallucinations (visual, auditory or tactile), fever, sweating and tachycardia. There is a mortality of 10%.

Alcoholic hallucinosis is a rare condition where hallucinations, usually auditory, occur in clear consciousness.

Morbid jealousy or the *Othello syndrome* involves firmly held delusions of a partner's infidelity. The alcoholic may search his partner's belongings for signs of infidelity or interrogate them about their daily activities. Under continual pressure unwise partners may confess to an infidelity that they have not committed. Unfortunately, such an admission of guilt may provoke a violent assault or even murder. Even in partners who continue to maintain their innocence geographical separation may be necessary to save their lives.

Depression and suicide are more common amongst alcoholics. Suicide is made more likely because of all the social consequences of alcohol abuse, e.g. job loss and divorce, and also because of the disinhibiting effect of alcohol. Depression often resolves without antidepressants once the alcoholic stops drinking.

Cognitive decline secondary to alcohol toxicity, trauma and thiamine deficiency may lead to difficulty on cognitive testing. Short-term recall, narrowness of thinking and impairment of visuospatial awareness are common findings. A high proportion of alcoholics have cortical atrophy and ventricular enlargement on brain imaging. *Wernicke's encephalopathy* is an acute reaction to severe thiamine deficiency and is characterised by delirium, confabulation, memory impairment, ataxia, nystagmus and peripheral neuropathy. *The Korsakoff state* is a chronic form without the delirium. Some people classify the two together as *Wernicke-Korsakoff syndrome*. High dose thiamine replacement may help reverse some cognitive deficits.

Family consequences

- Childhood physical abuse.
- Childhood sexual abuse.
- Alcoholism and substance abuse.
- Adult depression.
- Foetal alcohol syndrome. Features include growth retardation, small head circumference, small eyes, flattened bridge of nose and mental retardation.

Consequences to society

Sixty per cent of convicts report alcohol problems. One-third of all drivers killed have excess alcohol in their blood.

As a consequence of offending behaviour such as sexual assault or drink driving, unrelated third parties may be psychologically damaged, e.g. through post-traumatic stress disorder or bereavement.

Side-effects of street drugs

Drug users will often deny to themselves and others that drugs have adverse consequences, but unfortunately they do, especially if from an impure source or rogue batch. Some of the common side-effects of street drugs are given in Table 8.3. Paradoxically, addicts may be at risk from unusually pure supplies of street drugs. Street heroin is often adulterated with other substances. A purer supply may mean that the addict uses too much and overdoses themselves unwittingly.

Treatment options for alcoholics

Options for alcoholism

The main aspect necessary for recovery is the will of the patient to conquer their alcohol problem. It may seem obvious to say that before the problem can be conquered it must be recognised, but alcohol problems often persist for a long time before the individual can accept that they have a problem. The alcoholic's tendency to use *projection* often means that the solution is seen as outside themselves and their recovery is seen as being the responsibility of external agencies. External agencies such as hospitals can assist in detoxification and specialist hostels can provide support in terms of shelter and encouragement, but the fundamental change in behaviour required is ultimately the responsibility of the addict. Involving family members as co-therapists is often useful and ongoing support from self-help and other groups is vital.

Medical help for alcoholics

In detoxification or withdrawal regimes, benzodiazepines can be useful in allaying withdrawal symptoms and raising the fit threshold. On coming into hospital a regular, high dose of benzodiazepines is given and over the next week or so is gradually reduced. The object is to avoid a full blown alcohol withdrawal syndrome, with all the dangers that this entails. Thiamine and multivitamin supplements may be needed to prevent the Wernicke-Korsakoff syndrome. Attention to hydration, electrolyte and glucose balance and exclusion of infection is important. Specific advice on physical consequences of alcoholism may be necessary. Psychological problems may require onward referral. In the long-term treatment of alcoholics there is sometimes use of a drug called disulfiram which produces an adverse reaction if the taker drinks alcohol. The reaction involves flushing, nausea, headache, tachycardia, difficulty in breathing and hypotension.

Medical treatment options for drug addicts

Withdrawal or maintenance programmes for heroin addicts often use the opiate substitute methadone. In these programmes methadone is supplied in a

Table 8.3 Street drugs, methods of use, side-effects and origins

Drug	Drug route	Side-effects	Source
Cocaine and Crack	Sniffed, smoked, injected	Tachycardia, hypertension, insomnia, anorexia, agitation, hyperthermia, depression, persecutory delusions, hallucinations, fits, death	Peru, Bolivia, Colombia
Amphetamines	Oral, injected	Paranoia, depression, hypomania psychotic phenomena, tachycardia, other cardiac arrhythmias, hypertension, diuresis, insomnia, death	Laboratories in UK, Netherlands, Scandinavia and US
Benzodiazepines	Oral, injected	Respiratory depression, ataxia, disorientation, unconsciousness	Public houses, street sources, prescriptions
Heroin and methadone	Oral and injected (methadone), Sniffed, injected, smoked (heroin)	Respiratory depression, constipation, nausea, clammy skin, pupil constriction, coma	Iran, Pakistan, Afghanistan, Burma, Thailand, Laos, Mexico, Guatemala, Colombia
Lysergic acid (LSD)	Oral	Illusions and hallucinations, altered body perception, dissociative experiences, lability of mood, psychotic illnesses, flashback phenomena	USA and Netherlands
Psilocybin	Oral (teas made from magic mushrooms)	Tachycardia, hypertension, pupillary dilatation, visual illusions and hallucinations, nausea and stomach pains	Woodland areas
Cannabis	Oral	Fatigue, apathy, impaired memory and attention, bronchitis, carcinogenic	A bushy, easily cultivated, plant found worldwide. Pakistan, Morocco, Nigeria and Jamaica
MDMA (Ecstasy)	Oral — tablets	Tachycardia, pupillary dilatation, nausea, hyperthermia and muscle breakdown, disorientation, psychotic states, memory deficits, depression, fits, death	Netherlands and Belgium, Eastern Europe
Steroids	Oral, injected	Fatigue, aggression, liver and kidney damage, hypertension, sterility, insomnia, depression, paranoid psychoses, cardiac failure, death	Gymnasia, street sources
Solvents	Inhaled	Cardiac arrhythmias, suffocation, fires, ataxia, slurred speech, nausea, hallucinations, coma, death	Hardware stores and supermarkets

reducing course over several weeks or months, or in maintenance programmes is prescribed almost indefinitely. Advantages of such programmes include medical supervision, clean needles, pure drugs and a reduced local crime rate. Disadvantages include the addictivity of methadone and the selling on of methadone, or the 'topping-up' of pre-scribed sources with other street drugs by the addict. Naltrexone is an oral long-acting antagonist which the detoxified addict can take. Further drug abuse is not associated with any effect because of the antagonism, thereby eliminating any reward effect. Drug-rehabilitation units and hostels are available, but rare.

Withdrawal from amphetamines or other stimulants can be aided by the use of tricyclic antidepressants. Benzodiazepine addiction can be managed by switching the addict onto a longer acting compound and gradually withdrawing this over weeks or months.

CASE HISTORY 1

A 34-year-old married man called Nicholas was brought to hospital by ambulance. His colleagues at the college where he worked as a librarian had found him slumped over a desk in the library archives. He had drunk almost the whole contents of a bottle of vodka. He had been sick everywhere, but he was also nearly unconscious. He was admitted to a medical ward and seen the next day by the duty psychiatrist who noticed that Nicholas had a clammy handshake, was shaking all over and looked very sweaty. Whilst he was talking Nicholas kept wringing his hands and seemed very anxious. He cried twice during the interview.

He gave a history of heavy drinking for the past 6 months, ever since his supervisor at work had set certain targets for his department. The drinking had caused many arguments with his wife, whom he had hit twice. He said that this was 'out of character' and 'because of the drink'. His wife was an 'unforgiving and hard' woman and had left him, taking their two children with her. He had tried to phone her at her mother's house, but the family had had the telephone number changed. Feeling very sorry for himself, Nicholas had bought a bottle of vodka intending to drink it all at work and kill himself through alcoholic self-poisoning. The psychiatrist enquired about various other symptoms and learnt that Nicholas had early morning wakening, loss of appetite and had been having memory problems. He kept forgetting what had happened the day before.

How would you assess this man further?

He needs to have a full history taken, a mental state examination, particularly cognitive function, a physical examination, some physical investigations and a corroborative history.

What cognitive tests would you be most interested in?

Orientation and, providing that his attention and concentration is adequate, tests of short-term memory such as the Doctor's name, three objects (apple, table, chair) and a seven component name and address. It might be worth investigating whether he gets repeatedly lost on the ward, because visual/spatial memory is often impaired. The importance of such tests is to exclude delirium (by testing orientation) and to exclude a Korsakoff state (short-term memory). He admits to some memory problems. Forgetting the previous day's events is sometimes called *palimpsest*.

What would the immediate management of this man be?

He is in alcohol withdrawal (he is anxious and sweating, has a tremor and may well also have pupillary dilatation and tachycardia). Not only is the withdrawal unpleasant but there is also a risk of convulsions as the epileptic threshold is reduced. A detoxification regime is required using reducing doses of a benzodiazepine such as chlordiazepoxide. You would also need to exclude metabolite disturbances and coexisting infection.

CASE HISTORY 2

Kevin was 18 when he arrived as a new patient at the health centre. He claimed that he had just moved into the area and needed to register with a new family doctor. He seemed very keen to see the doctor that day, but would not explain why to the receptionist and was rude to her when she asked a second time. When he did see the new doctor he gave a history of drug abuse since the age of 13, when he had first experimented with school friends sniffing glue out of plastic bags. When one of his friends died from experimenting with sniffing butane, Kevin moved onto 'safer' drugs. For a few years he smoked cannabis, but latterly had been injecting heroin. His mother had thrown him out of her house. He had spent 6 months in jail. Even so he continued to burgle houses and steal cars to fund his habit.

He said that he was very keen to come off

drugs 'once and for all' and that he needed the doctor to prescribe a course of intravenous methadone to help him come off heroin. When the doctor said that he referred all his patients with drug problems to the regional drug clinic Kevin became very abusive, to the doctor's surprise. Kevin accused the doctor of being suspicious and then broke down into tears of frustration as he pleaded with the doctor to 'give him a break'. He apologised for his earlier anger. The doctor reached for his prescription pad, but at that moment the phone rang. It was the health centre receptionist. She had checked Kevin's details and the address he had given was false. When the doctor turned to confront Kevin with this he found that Kevin had already gone.

What feelings are aroused in health professionals by such patients?

Although carers may start out with good intentions and high ideals they run the risk of becoming cynical when faced with patients like Kevin who will cheat and thieve to fulfil their cravings. Finally, though, Kevin is deceiving himself more than anyone else.

The negative feelings engendered by such patients need to be acknowledged. If carers deny them they deceive themselves and may be fooled into making decisions which they think are justifiable, but are in fact motivated more by cynicism and dislike. Such negative feelings may lead carers to ignore vital information. For example, a doctor may fail to examine an unconscious patient properly in the mistaken belief that they *are* merely drunk when, in fact, they are drunk but they also have a skull fracture. Furthermore, it is important to realise that some addicts do mean what they say and can carry out their promises to reform. Some studies show that addicts are best helped by care and encouragement from staff with high motivation.

LEARNING POINTS

Addiction

- *Tolerance* implies that repeated use of the drug produces less effect for the same dose.
- *Dependence* may be physical or psychological and implies that without the drug the addict suffers physical or psychological symptoms in a *withdrawal syndrome.*
- Substance abuse is more common in men than women.
- The main thing necessary for long-term recovery is the will of the patient to conquer their addiction.
- Alcoholism is linked to a 15% lifetime risk of suicide.
- Ten per cent of alcoholics have had fits.
- *Delirium tremens* is an acute confusional state which may occur 24–96 hours after stopping drinking. Symptoms include marked tremor, restlessness, disorientation, illusions and hallucinations, fever, sweating and tachycardia. There is a mortality of 10%.
- In general hospitals 20–30% of all male admissions and 5–10% of all female admissions are probably heavy drinkers.
- Addiction is not confined to any single portion of society and is endemic throughout the world.
- Street drug use is rising and drug users are getting younger. It is difficult to control access to addictive substances such as solvents, which are freely available. Small laboratories are easily set up to create supplies of crack cocaine, LSD, amphetamines and ecstasy. In view of all drugs' ready availability, combating drug abuse requires health education which changes people's attitudes towards drugs and alcohol.
- Although most alcohol and drug use does not bring people into contact with psychiatry, both put people at increased risk of affective disorders, psychotic disorders and suicide.

Self-assessment

MCQs

1 Features of the chronic Korsakoff syndrome include:
   a delirium
   b anterograde amnesia
   c confabulation
   d psychotic symptoms
   e vertical nystagmus

2 Benzodiazepine withdrawal may produce:
   a tremor
   b insomnia

c anxiety
d convulsions
e muscle fasciculation

3 Methadone:
  a is a benzodiazepine
  b can be prescribed intravenously
  c has a shorter half-life than heroin
  d may induce vomiting
  e is not excreted in breast milk

4 Clinical features of chronic opiate dependence include:
  a dilated pupils
  b tremor
  c chronic tiredness
  d constipation
  e impotence

Short answer questions

1 What are the principles underlying treatment of someone with delirium tremens?
2 What are the clinical features of solvent abuse?
3 What are the effects and side-effects of amphetamine abuse?

MCQ answers

1 a = F, b = T, c = T, d = F, e = F
2 All true
3 a = F, b = T, c = F, d = T, e = F
4 a = F, b = T, c = T, d = T, e = T

Explorations

Sources listed in the 'Further reading and reference' section will help you with the following:

Links with public health

Look at the data in Table 8.4 about alcohol consumption and cirrhosis of the liver. What conclusions can you draw?

Links with medicine

What are the long-term physical consequences of alcohol dependence? How might these consequences fit in with psychological problems such as jealousy, memory problems and delirium? What physical investigations could be used to identify alcohol abusers in general medical practice?

Links with general practice

What evidence is there that screening questionnaires (such as those in Table 8.5) are useful in identifying alcoholics in general practice?

Further reading and references

CHICK J 1987 Early intervention in the general hospital. In: Stockwell T, Clement S (eds) Helping the problem drinker. Croom Helm, London

CHICK J 1992 Doctors with emotional problems: how can they be helped? In: Hawton K, Cowen P (eds) Dilemmas in the management of psychiatric patients. Oxford University Press, Oxford

US NATIONAL INSTITUTE of JUSTICE 1991 Research in action: drug use forecasting. US Department of Justice, Washington

MAYFIELD D, McLEOD G, HALL P 1974 The CAGE questionnaire: validation of a new alcoholism screening instrument. American Journal of Psychiatry 131: 1121–1123

POKORNY A D, MILLER B A, KAPLAN H B 1972 The brief MAST: a shortened version of the Michigan alcohol-

Table 8.4   National trends in alcohol consumption and deaths/100 000 from liver cirrhosis (WHO Statistics 1991 and 1974–1983)

Country	Alcohol consumed (litres per adult)					Liver cirrhosis (deaths/100 000)	
	1970	1975	1980	1984	1989	1974	1989
France	19.6	18.6	14.8	14.2	13.4	32.8	19.9
GDR	6.3	8.2	9.7	13.3	11.1	12.5	19.6
USA	6.8	7.9	8.7	7.9	7.5	15.8	10.8
Finland	4.5	6.7	6.4	6.6	7.6	5.5	9.8

ism screening test. American Journal of Psychiatry 129: 342–345

RAY O, KSIR C 1993 Drugs, society and human behaviour, 6th edn. Mosby, St. Louis

WRIGHT J D, PEARL L 1990 Knowledge and experience of young people regarding drug abuse 1969–1989. British Medical Journal 300: 99–103

Table 8.5 The CAGE and MAST questionnaires. The CAGE questions (Mayfield et al., 1974) are an example of a validated screening instrument for alcoholism: two positive answers on the CAGE are strongly suggestive of alcoholism. The shortened Michigan Alcoholism Screening Test (MAST) is a series of 10 alternative questions (Pokorny et al., 1972). To score the brief MAST, you score 2 for a negative answer to the first and second questions, and for positive answers to the remainder you score either 5 or 2. For question 3, yes = 5, for question 4, yes = 2. For questions 5, 6, 7, 8, 9 and 10, score 2, 2, 2, 5, 5 and 2 respectively for positive answers. A score above 18 indicates severe problems. Most non-alcoholics score less than 5.

CAGE questionnaire

- **C** Have you ever felt you should CUT down on your drinking?
- **A** Have people ANNOYED you by criticising your drinking?
- **G** Have you ever felt bad or GUILTY about your drinking?
- **E** Have you ever had a drink first thing in the morning to steady your nerves or get rid of a hang-over (eye-opener)?

MAST questionnaire

- Do you feel you are a normal drinker?
- Do friends or relatives think you are a normal drinker?
- Have you ever attended a meeting of Alcoholics Anonymous (AA)?
- Have you ever lost friends or girl/boyfriends because of drinking?
- Have you ever got into trouble at work because of drinking?
- Have you ever neglected your obligations, your family, your work for more than 2 days in a row because you were drinking?
- Have you ever had delirium tremens (DTs), severe shaking, heard voices or seen things that weren't there after heavy drinking?
- Have you ever been in a hospital because of your drinking?
- Have you ever been arrested for drunk driving or driving after drinking?

Addiction in literature

AMIS K W 1969 The Green Man
DE QUINCEY T 1821 Confessions of an English Opium Eater
VONNEGUT M 1975 The Eden Express

Resources

Action on Addiction,
York House,
199, Westminster House,
London SE1 7UT
Tel: 0171 261 1333

Alcohol Concern,
275 Gray's Inn Road,
London WC1X 8QF
Tel: 0171 833 3471

Alcoholics Anonymous,
P O Box 1,
Stonebow House,
Stonebow,
York Y01 2NJ

Drugline Ltd.,
9a Brockley Cross,
Brockley,
London SE4 2AB
Tel: 0181 692 4975

Families Anonymous,
Room 8,
650 Holloway Road,
London N19 3NU
Tel: 0171 281 8889

Release,
169 Commercial Street,
London E1 6BW
Tel: 0171 377 5905

Turning Point,
CAP House,
9/12 Long Lane,
London EC1A 9HA

9

Personality

Every individual's personality is unique. Personality is a combination of biological temperament, willingness to explore and socialise, intelligence, education and accumulated experience in reaction to life events. Personality may dictate how people react to illness. Some personalities are so different to others that they are sometimes called personality disorders. The behaviour of people with extreme personalities may lead to them harming themselves or others.

Contents

Personality development and types

Personality and the neonate

If you listen to mothers describing their children they will often tell you how each pregnancy had its own characteristics and how even at birth each child differed in some way from its siblings. Some babies seem very active in the womb and react to their mother's behaviour, others seem relatively inactive. At birth some babies are relatively alert and excitable, others are more stolid. Obviously some of these stories are altered by circumstance over the years to explain the temperament or character of the child, 'he always was outgoing — how he made his voice heard when he was born!' and suffer from the problems of retrospective recall. And some events cloud 'observations' of neonatal 'character', for instance if pain relief is given to the mother in labour, the neonate may have depressed levels of consciousness. However, there is work to suggest biological differences in excitability and even learning ability (in terms of habituation to stimuli) in embryos and neonates. These biological differences probably form the core of personality.

Mother and child

The newborn baby and his or her mother react and adapt to each other. The components and effect of this dyadic relationship are difficult to disentangle because there are symbiotic needs and behaviours involved. People often think that the needs are wholly the baby's and that the parent is the sole provider. However, the mother has subtle emotional needs too, and the growing baby may or may not be able to fulfil these. The baby rewards the mother's care by, say, becoming quiet or content when fed; the older infant is able to reward behaviour it likes by smiles or vocalisations.

There is an *attachment* between mother and child which may be secure or insecure. The secure infant will be able to make small explorations away from the mother. The insecure infant will cling and protest at any actual or threatened separation from mother. After necessary separations the secure infant will (after some protest) resume its secure behaviour whilst the insecure infant will continue to express its distress and anxiety that its mother will disappear again. The child forms an internal work-ing model of such relationships. Later in life when there are changing circumstances in any relationship (such as separation or loss) this internal working model (stable or unstable) may be evoked.

Jung

How outgoing people are and how easily they form relationships are reflected in Carl Jung's concepts of *extraversion* and *introversion*. Extraverts are people who socialise easily and enjoy company. They are the explorers of life, seeking out new experiences and making their views known. Introverts prefer their own company or the company of a restricted band of close friends. They tend to be loners, conservative in their tastes and often keeping their ideas to themselves.

Freud

Sigmund Freud's model of personality was that there were three distinct components: the id, the ego and the superego. The id is that portion which is driven by various forces such as hunger or sexual desire. Such imperatives create a tension which can only be discharged once the desired object, e.g. food or sex, is obtained. The ego is that rational part of the personality which can plan out how to achieve the id's object. The superego is that part which judges the relative merits of the individual's behaviour in terms of conscience. The personality is, therefore, derived from an interaction between the id, ego and superego. Substance abusers are largely id driven; everything is directed towards satisfying an intense craving. Obsessional people are directed by their superegos which demand a strict adherence to rules.

Sigmund Freud (1856–1939) and his daughter Anna (1895–1982) also described various psychological defence mechanisms used by the individual to minimise their own psychological discomfort or tension (see Table 9.1). Everybody uses some of these defences to some extent at one time. However, when one or two defence mechanisms are used almost exclusively the individual may run into problems. Substance abusers often over–use denial and projection. They deny the severity of their drug problem to themselves and often project the reasons for their behaviour onto others: 'I need this drink

Table 9.1 Psychological defence mechanisms

- **Repression.** The person's own uncomfortable or unbearable ideas or feelings (such as aggression or sexual desires) are repressed from the conscious mind into the unconscious.
- **Denial.** In denial the individual often does not personally accept unpleasant thoughts, memories or emotions that they have. This is different to lying, where the person is consciously aware of what the truth is but is deceiving someone else. In denial there is a deception of the conscious self in order to avoid psychological pain. For instance, a patient, told of a terminal diagnosis, may appear to fail to take in the information.
- **Projection.** In projection the person attributes undesirable aspects of the self to other people, e.g. the alcoholic who blames his habit on the actions of others, or the thug who blames his own bad luck or incompetence on someone from a persecuted minority.
- **Splitting.** In splitting there is a tendency to see others in either a very good or a very bad light, the possibility that another may have a mixture of traits is not held. Other people are frequently idealised at first only to be cast down as fallen idols when they do not fit in with the person's needs or desires.
- **Displacement.** In displacement, feelings, usually of anger or fear, are displaced from one person or thing to another. So, for instance, a man who feels anger towards his supervisor may 'take it out' on his wife when they meet for dinner, unaware of the fact that his anger is more about his boss than his wife, who may be blameless.
- **Rationalisation.** After the event reasoning is used to justify actions and reduce hurt. The person who fails to attend a difficult appointment may justify his failure to himself on spurious grounds, e.g. I just missed the right bus. The rationalisation may have an element of truth, but can be confronted. Maybe the person that missed the bus did not want to get to the bus stop early enough.
- **Reaction formation.** Where people with various feelings develop opposite attitudes, e.g. people who feel chaotic and dirty become obsessionally tidy and clean, or people who have a need to be cared for or a fear of decay and death become carers or healers.
- **Sublimation.** Where a person uses the tension produced by an inner conflict to create, e.g. in writing or painting.

because my wife is so awful. It's her fault that I drink.'

Repressed ideas or memories may sometimes be coded in dreams in a symbolic way. Sigmund Freud often talked with his patients about their dreams to help them gain a better understanding of themselves and their inner fantasies and feelings.

Adler

Alfred Adler (1870–1937) said that there were four basic styles of coping with life's problems and that people tended to use one style in particular and that this helped define their personality type. The four types were the *dominant* type who rules without regard for others, the *getting* type who gets other people to solve their problems for them, the *avoiding* type who avoids difficulties and makes no attempt to face problems, and the *socially useful* type who co–operates with others and acts in accordance with their interests.

Adler was particularly interested in family structure and its effects on the development of the personality. First-borns, second-borns, youngest children and only children all have certain characteristics that depend upon their birth order. For instance, first borns receive undivided parental attention until 'dethroned' by the arrival of the second-born. Their life is often dominated from then on by a battle to regain supremacy. Younger siblings have to develop language and motor skills quickly to compete with their elders. An only child generally does not learn to share and compete as well as a child with siblings.

Behaviour and personality

It is difficult to disentangle behaviour from personality. Learning theory suggests that some people behave in certain ways because they keep receiving rewards for that kind of behaviour. The reward reinforces the behaviour. For people who find social situations very stressful, staying on their own provides a reward (the absence of anxiety) which reinforces their solitude. There is a continual feedback between the individual and the environment, much in the same way that in early life there is a continual feedback between the infant and his or her temperament and mother.

Cattell and trait theory

Instead of looking at people and classifying them into different types, another way of looking at the problem is to say that all personalities are different, but that some people have various traits to a greater or lesser extent. So, for example, one person may have strong obsessional traits.

Raymond Cattell, an English trait theorist born in 1905, believed that different people have various personality factors all acting to a different degree. Over two decades he analysed various traits using factor analysis and identified 16 so-called *source* traits which form the core of the Sixteen Personality Factor (16PF) Questionnaire. The traits are presented in Table 9.2.

Maslow

Abraham Maslow (1908–1970) described various needs that people have, and put them into a hierarchy (see Fig. 9.1). He also reversed the kind of thinking that lay behind many descriptions of personality types and traits and, instead of looking for pathology, looked for ideals of personality that people could aspire to. He called the ideal personality type a *self-actualising* personality. Self-actualisation is the realisation or fulfilment of potentials and capabilities. Such personalities are rare (less than 1% of the population) and have certain characteristics described in Figure 9.1.

Table 9.2 Cattell's 16 personality factors

Factor	A person with a low score on this factor is described as:	A person with a high score on this factor is described as:
A	Reserved	Outgoing
B	Less intelligent	More intelligent
C	Affected by feelings	Emotionally stable
E	Submissive	Dominant
F	Serious	Happy-go-lucky
G	Expedient	Conscientious
H	Timid	Venturesome
I	Toughminded	Sensitive
L	Trusting	Suspicious
M	Practical	Imaginative
N	Forthright	Shrewd
O	Self-assured	Apprehensive
Q_1	Conservative	Experimenting
Q_2	Group-dependent	Self-sufficient
Q_3	Uncontrolled	Controlled
Q_4	Relaxed	Tense

Personality disorders

Some people dislike the term 'personality disorder', because it can be used as an unpleasant label for people who are not likeable and who are often denied help. It implies that there are 'normal' personalities (you and I) and 'abnormal' personalities (them). In fact, there is probably a spectrum of personalities, not just two categories of normal and abnormal. Although the term personality disorders

Hierarchy of needs

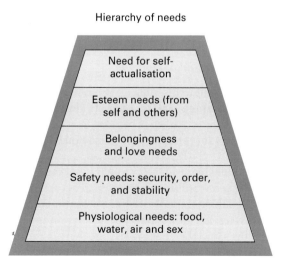

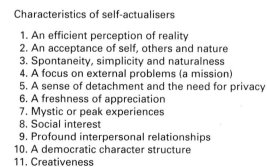

Characteristics of self-actualisers

1. An efficient perception of reality
2. An acceptance of self, others and nature
3. Spontaneity, simplicity and naturalness
4. A focus on external problems (a mission)
5. A sense of detachment and the need for privacy
6. A freshness of appreciation
7. Mystic or peak experiences
8. Social interest
9. Profound interpersonal relationships
10. A democratic character structure
11. Creativeness
12. Resistance to enculturation

Fig. 9.1 Abraham Maslow's hierarchy of needs and the characteristics of self-actualisers.

is awkward, there are sometimes extreme characters who need some description and so the term is used. Personality disorders are, therefore, extreme personalities who persistently behave in ways that are detrimental to themselves, to others or to society as a whole. Before you could use the term about someone you would need to be sure that their personality was developed as far as it could be (i.e. that they were not children), that your assessment was thorough (including an informant history) and that the abnormal behaviours were not because of psychological or organic illness (e.g. hypomania or frontal lobe damage).

Types of personality disorder

A *dissocial* or *sociopathic* personality is one where there is a callous lack of concern for the feelings of others, a persistent and irresponsible disregard for social norms and rules, difficulty in maintaining relationships and an inability to learn from experience, particularly punishment. Sociopaths may, therefore, be persistent offenders who behave without regard to their victims' feelings. Conduct disorder in childhood may precede adult dissocial behaviour.

An *obsessional* or *anankastic* personality is one where there is excessive caution and a slavish attention to detail, order, timetables and rules. Colleagues of such people may be infuriated by their perfectionism and slowness. When urged to hurry or to cut corners the anankastic individual can resort to stubbornness.

A *dependent* personality is one where the individual gets other people to make decisions on their behalf. They comply with others' wishes to an extreme degree and feel helpless when alone. A fear of abandonment allows certain people to disregard their best interests and such dependent people often seem to settle in relationships where their partner is excessively dominant or cruel.

A *schizoid* personality is perceived by others as being emotionally cold and unable to express warm feelings. They seem indifferent to close, sexual relationships and even friendships with others. Often such people do not even have one close friend. As loners they seem to have an intense preoccupation with their own fantasies and ideas.

A *paranoid* personality is markedly sensitive to minor setbacks. They bear grudges and will not forgive injuries or slights. Their outlook on the world tends to colour their relationships with others and they will perceive criticism or rebuffs where none was intended. Their focus on themselves because they feel that everyone thinks more about them than they actually do is suggestive of a certain self-importance. Such people may be suspicious, jealous of their rights (and consequently litigious) or jealous of the sexual fidelity of their partners. They will prefer explanations of events which incorporate the notion of a 'conspiracy' against them or parts of society.

A *borderline or emotionally unstable* personality is often affected by bursts of intense emotion, such as anger, and may act impulsively to self-harm, e.g. cutting. There is a sense of confusion about identity, a tendency to have brief, intense and unstable relationships, a tendency to dissociate from their true feelings and to use defence mechanisms like *splitting* and *projection*. A childhood history of sexual abuse is often found. Sometimes brief psychotic experiences occur and require medication.

Personality disorders are variants of personality and, since all personalities can be affected by illness, it is very important to realise that people with personality disorders may have coexisting mental or physical disorders which may need treatment.

CASE HISTORY 1

Rachel had been seeing psychiatrists since the age of 15. Her mother, unable to cope with her behaviour, threw her out when she was aged 18. At the age of 20 she was taken to hospital with her seventh paracetamol overdose. The duty psychiatrist who saw her on a medical ward noticed that her forearms were so scarred from repeated cutting that they were more scar tissue than skin.

Rachel was unwilling to give a history to the doctor, but from her thick file of notes the psychiatrist noted several details about her past.

Rachel's father had left home when she was 7. Up to that age Rachel could only remember her parents repeated rows and the fact that she lived in fear of her father beating her. Her mother married again when Rachel was 10. Rachel suffered sexual abuse at the hands of her stepfather. When her mother learnt about the abuse she accused Rachel of seducing her new husband, but she did insist on a divorce from him for which Rachel was grateful.

At the age of 13 Rachel had her first sexual intercourse with an 18-year-old fairground worker. She left home to stay with him in a caravan, but returned home 3 weeks later. She began drinking heavily at the age of 14 and started having a series of affairs with older men. Most of the affairs were short-lived. The longest time that she saw anyone was two months. At the age of 15 she took an overdose of her mother's antidepressants and saw her first psychiatrist.

What features about Rachel's history suggest an abnormal personality?

There is a long history of deliberate self-harm, impulsive behaviour — alcohol abuse and inappropriate sexual liaisons — and unstable relationships. The behaviours assume a repeating pattern. Presumably at the start of each sexual relationship Rachel sees the other as desirable in some way, but very soon they are rejected, possibly because they are seen in a suddenly negative light. This might suggest the use of *splitting* as a defence mechanism. Overall there are features suggestive of a borderline personality disorder.

What is there about Rachel's early life which may explain some of her personality and behaviour?

Nearly all her relationships are inconsistent ones, either because of others' actions or her own. Her parents' relationship was unstable and ended in failure at a critical point in her development. Children often blame themselves if their parents split up. More undeserved blame was laid at Rachel's door by her mother after her second marriage failed. In Rachel's position people often take the blame on board and feel profoundly guilty; they are indeed a bad person. They see the people around them as either good or bad and view themselves in the same unforgiving way. Rachel may feel good about herself sometimes, but this is always followed by feelings of guilt and badness. In helping such people it is difficult not to be sucked into being as inconsistent as previous figures in their

life. Consistency is something to be aimed for in terms of management. A long-term therapeutic relationship can help where sessions with the same person are regularly, but not necessarily frequently, given. Predictably, such therapy will revolve around issues of guilt, persecution and fear of rejection.

CASE HISTORY 2

Miss Arbuthnot, 60, called her family doctor out to see her one weekend. She had never called a doctor out before. In fact she had not seen a doctor in 20 years. She was embarrassed at having to do so, but had developed a chest infection and was feeling quite unwell.

Her family doctor was concerned that Miss Arbuthnot had pneumonia and had no one to care for her during her illness. She rejected his offer to arrange a hospital admission, because she could not face 'a ward full of strangers'. She would take anything he prescribed for her, but she would not leave her home nor allow any 'stranger' in to give her help. For Miss Arbuthnot a 'stranger' was just about anybody. Even her closest neighbours were 'strangers'. She had only called the doctor because she felt desperate. It was clear that she resented his probing questions. It seemed that she had not one friend in the world. She occasionally went out to a local church and sat at the very back on her own. She fled if anyone asked her to stay for coffee after the service. She shopped in the supermarket to avoid conversation. All her relatives had died, but it seemed that they were never a close family. She had worked briefly in insurance as 'a girl', but found people to be 'busybodies'. She had never had a boyfriend, although someone had asked her out, once. Her hobbies included listening to the music of Liszt and Chopin and reading the works of Marx and Engels.

She did not appear to be depressed, demented or psychotic and the doctor was unable to persuade her to go to hospital. Reluctantly he gave her some antibiotics and said he would return in a few days. She replied that he should not do this and that she would call if she needed to see him again. Having ushered the doctor out of her house she closed the front door and sighed with relief.

What features suggest an abnormal personality?

This lady has virtually no relationships at all beyond the superficial ones that are essential to daily transactions such as going to the supermarket. She avoids all deeper contact. There is no friendship or sexual relationship in her life. Such avoidant behaviour has characterised her behaviour all through her life. Even the superficial contact with a family doctor is resented. Her only interests are solitary ones. She could be described as a schizoid personality. Helping her, as the family doctor found, would be an uphill struggle unless she herself desired to change.

LEARNING POINTS

Personality

- There are numerous theories of personality based on different types or traits. Extraversion and introversion are two personality types often referred to and were first described by Carl Jung.
- Sigmund Freud described the personality as an interaction between id, ego and superego. He and his daughter also defined various defence mechanisms such as denial, projection, splitting and sublimation.
- Dreams may sometimes highlight internal conflicts and repressed material in symbolic form.
- Personality disordered individuals have extreme personalties and repeatedly behave in ways that are detrimental to themselves, the people around them and/or society.
- *Dissocial* or *sociopathic* personality disorder involves a callous lack of concern for others' feelings, difficulty in maintaining relationships and an inability to learn from experience. This may lead to sufferers becoming persistent offenders.
- *Obsessional* or *anankastic* personality disorder involves excessive caution and slavish attention to detail, perfectionism, stubbornness and slowness.
- *Dependent* personality disorder involves someone getting other people to make decisions on their behalf and complying with others' wishes to the detriment of the self because of a fear of abandonment.
- *Schizoid* personality disorder involves emotional coldness and an inability to express warm feelings. Close, sexual relationships and friendships are avoided and there is a preoccupation with fantasies and ideas.

- *Paranoid* personality disorder sufferers are suspicious, bear grudges and will not forgive injuries or slights, often where none was actually intended. Their focus on themselves is suggestive of a certain self-importance.
- *Borderline* personality disorder sufferers have bursts of intense emotion, like anger. They may act impulsively to harm themselves. There is confusion about their own identity, dissociation from their true feelings and the frequent use of defence mechanisms like *splitting* and *projection*.
- Personality disorders may have coexisting mental or physical disorders needing treatment.

Self-assessment

MCQs

1 Psychological defence mechanisms include:
  a denial
  b projection
  c displacement
  d materialism
  e mobilisation

2 Recognised personality traits include:
  a obsessionality
  b conscientiousness
  c suspiciousness
  d openness
  e submissiveness

Essays

1 Describe the id, the ego and the superego. How do they work together to determine personality and behaviour?
2 What is the unconscious? How do we know whether there is an unconscious or not?
3 What is personality and how does it develop?
4 Describe how people with disordered personalities present to medical care.

MCQ answers

1 a = T, b = T, c = T, d = F, e = F
2 All true

Explorations

Sources listed in the Further reading and reference section will help you with the following.

Links with psychology

1 Find out about the *16 Personality Factor Questionnaire* and the *Myers–Briggs Type Indicator*. Look at the personality types or factors that they use. Which category or categories do you think might fit you best? What other personality tests are there? What research has been done to demonstrate their scientific validity? How reliable are they? What are they used for in society?

2 Study the list of psychological defence mechanisms. Can you think of examples from your own experience that might illustrate each mechanism? Do you recognise any of the mechanisms in yourself?

Links with genetics

What evidence is there to suggest that personality has an inherited basis rather than being solely a product of environment and upbringing? What kind of studies have been or could be done to establish the genetic contribution?

Further reading and references

BOWLBY J 1979 The making and breaking of affectional bonds. Tavistock, London

EPTING F R 1984 Personal construct counselling and psychotherapy. Wiley, New York

ERIKSON E H 1968 Identity: youth and crisis. Norton, New York

GAY P 1988 Freud: a life for our time. Norton, New York

JUNG C G 1961 Memories, dreams and reflections. Vintage Books, New York

MASLOW A H 1970 Motivation and personality, 2nd edn. Harper & Row, New York

MCCAULEY M H 1990 The Myers–Briggs type indicator: a measure for individuals and groups. Measurement and evaluation in counselling and development **22**: 181–195

PLOMIN R 1990 Nature and nurture: an introduction to human behavioural genetics. Brooks Cole, Pacific Grove, CA

ROAZEN P 1975 Freud and his followers. Knopf, New York

SAUNDERS F 1991 Mother's light, daughter's journey: Katharine and Isabel. Consulting Psychologists Press, Palo Alto, CA

WORLD HEALTH ORGANIZATION 1992 The ICD–10 classification of mental and behavioural disorders. F60–F69 Disorders of adult personality and behaviour. World Health Organization, Geneva, p. 198–224

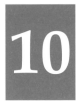

10

Child and adolescent psychiatry

Children with psychological problems are dependent on others, such as parents or teachers, to recognise their distress and arrange help for them. It is likely that much of this psychological distress is overlooked. Child psychiatrists differ in their practice from adult psychiatrists in three ways. Firstly, they must take into account the developmental stage that the child has reached. Secondly, the family and their stage in the family life cycle must be considered. Finally, child psychiatrists tend to rely on psychological methods of treatment rather than physical methods.

Contents

Psychological disorders in children

Some disorders may occur in children in forms that are similar to adults, e.g. phobias and obsessive compulsive disorder, but generally diagnoses in child psychiatry are less precise and are often formulated in terms of family or other problems.

Some diagnostic terms are specific to childhood. *Hyperkinetic disorders* involve overactivity, poor attention, poor concentration on tasks and disorganisation in *most* situations. Hyperkinetic disorders generally arise in the first 5 years of life. Hyperkinetic children are often impulsive, accident prone and may be seen as cheeky by adults and are unpopular with other children. Motor and language skills may be delayed. Hyperkinesis may be associated with a *conduct disorder*. Conduct disorders involve repeated antisocial, aggressive or defiant acts and are more severe than simple mischief or high spirits. Conduct disorders are more common in boys than girls. *Emotional disorders* are more common in girls than boys. The category of emotional disorders contains such problems as low mood, separation anxiety, phobic anxiety, social anxiety and sibling rivalry.

Other problems associated with childhood may include tics (involuntary, rapid, recurrent non-rhythmic motor movements) like eye-blinking and grimacing, non-organic enuresis (bedwetting) and non-organic encopresis (passage of faeces in inappropriate places). Tics are relatively common (10–20%) and usually resolve themselves. Rarely, tics may form part of Gilles de la Tourette syndrome and may respond to small doses of haloperidol. Non-organic enuresis occurs in 10% of 5 year olds, 4% of 8 year olds and 1% of 14 year olds. Management involves excluding organic problems (such as urinary tract infection), family assessment and behavioural therapies such as 'star charts' and 'bell and pad' alarms.

Treatment options

General practitioners and health visitors are important primary care resources and can help with advice and assessment.

Child psychiatrists are a relatively scarce resource, but they often work through child guidance clinics or special community mental health teams. Most of their work is done on an out-patient basis. In-patient facilities are rare nowadays. Child psychiatrists may use behavioural regimes, family and group therapy. Rarely, they may use physical treatments. Community mental health teams may also include community psychiatric nurses, child psychologists and special child social workers, who often have family therapy skills.

Educational psychologists are available within the school system and can help not only in identifying specific educational problems, e.g. dyslexia, but also in managing school related anxieties and may be vital in managing school refusal. Educational welfare officers also assist in managing school refusal and truancy.

The family life cycle

The family is like an organism which is born, lives, gives birth, ages and dies. A man and a woman from different families meet and form a permanent relationship, the nucleus of a new family. Their relationship together changes forever when a new child is born, and develops as more children are added. This growth phase of the family is followed by a plateau phase during which children are nurtured, trained and educated. One by one the children are ready to assume their own autonomous existence and leave the closeness of the family to begin their own separate lives. Contact may be maintained but the nuclear family is aging now and contracting as a result. Parents may react in a variety of ways to their offspring leaving them. Some parents may see themselves as desolated, others feel rewarded by the successful completion of their parental roles. Some children may never feel able to leave. Most do, however, and often seek out their own partners to renew the family life cycle.

Of course, the above cycle concerns a stereotyped version of a family. Not all families conform to this traditional Westernised pattern. Some families may exist altogether in an extended family. Some families may consist of a single parent and child.

CASE HISTORY 1

Tony, 12, was brought to the accident and emergency department by his father who had just stopped him trying to climb out of his bedroom window. The senior house officer in paediatrics noticed that Tony was unsteady on his feet and that his speech was slurred. Tony did not seem to know where he was. His father admonished him for giggling at the doctor and for pulling a rude face. His father said that when he had pulled Tony away from the window his son had talked about seeing a 'stairway to heaven'. There had been no previous contact with psychiatrists and Tony's general health had always been good.

What are the main problems?

Tony appears to be disorientated and disinhibited. It sounds as if he was misperceiving his environment at home too, because he was trying to climb out of the window in response to what sounds like a visual hallucination.

What could have caused these problems?

The key feature is the sudden onset of all these symptoms. The symptoms themselves have a strongly organic character: ataxia, slurred speech, visual hallucinations and disorientation. The sudden onset in a child may reflect a pyrexial illness or some epileptic phenomenon, but perhaps more likely in this case a drug-induced phenomenon. The doctor would need to know if Tony has been prescribed anything recently or whether he could have access to any prescribed medicines in the house. An overdose of a parent's tricyclic antidepressants could cause an equally sudden acute organic reaction. Street drugs may be to blame, and the parents might or might not know if these were available in Tony's school or neighbourhood. Similarly, they may or may not know whether Tony has in fact been experimenting with solvents or aerosol gas. Street drugs or solvent abuse can cause similar presentations. Trying to establish the cause of the reaction is important because of the physical consequences of some substances, e.g. arhythmias with solvents. If the psychotic reaction is caused by substance abuse, then it should subside fairly quickly, although some recreational drugs like LSD and ecstasy may have long term psychological effects.

| CASE HISTORY 2 |

Sue came to the doctor explaining about her two-year-old son, Mark. He would not sleep at night, she said, and now he was hyperactive and 'into everything' during the day.

'You'll probably think I'm just neurotic,' she said to the doctor. 'My husband does.' And indeed, as if to confound her, Mark sat quietly on his mother's lap throughout the entire interview.

The doctor eventually moved the interview round to talking about Sue's relationship with her husband since Mark's birth and also to discussing Sue's own sleeping pattern.

The doctor learnt that since the birth Sue and her husband, Richard, had 'drifted apart a bit' and that she focused her attention on Mark. She was very careful about what he ate, how he dressed and his 'untidiness' during play. Sue was not sleeping well and had early morning wakening. Instead of sleeping at 5 a.m. she went into Mark's room and busied herself getting his clothes ready for the morning. Mark, hearing his mother moving about his room, woke and began to play. During the day Sue felt irritable, frustrated, lonely and cried easily. When her husband came home from work she usually had a row with him because he took 'no interest' in his son.

What is the main problem according to Sue?

Mark is overactive and will not sleep at night.

How does the husband perceive the problem?

It is difficult to say because his opinion is reported by his wife, but it does sound as if there is some conflict between them. Sue says that her husband thinks she is 'neurotic'. It seems as if the arrival of Mark is related to an increasing distance between Sue and her husband.

How might the doctor perceive the problem?

If the doctor listens purely to what Sue says about Mark, he might think that some simple remedy to help Mark sleep at night would solve the problem. This *linear* thinking might lead some doctors to prescribe night sedation as a solution, with all the inherent problems of dependence that are associated.

There is a mismatch between what Sue reports and how Mark behaves in the surgery and this might direct the doctor towards other solutions. In particular it does sound as if Sue is herself unwell. Perhaps she has had an untreated postnatal depressive illness which is worsening all her problems. Is her nocturnal insomnia leading her to seek out contact with Mark and stopping him from sleeping at night? Treatment for Sue's depressive illness might be considered then, although Sue has already signalled that she does not accept her husband's suggestion that the problem lies with her. She feels that the solution is somewhere outside herself. If the doctor focused purely on this he might conflict with Sue, who might assume that he was 'blaming' her for the family's problems.

So, the problem cannot be represented by a simple *linear* cause and effect model. In other words, it is not Mark's overactivity or Sue's depression that is the single origin of all their problems. There is a *circular* process here partly because the whole family is involved. Figure 10.1 shows diagrams of how the family must have originally looked and how the arrival of Mark might have changed things. First there was a couple, and then a third person moved into the house and changed forever the relationship between husband and wife, leading to alternate distance and conflict. Sue's relationship with Mark may appear to be so strong to her husband that he feels excluded and is left to carp occasionally from the periphery of the family.

The family doctor might ask to see the whole family or ask a community psychiatric nurse to visit the family home to work with the family. Some simple suggestions to support the original family subsystem (the couple) could be made, for instance to leave Mark to sleep through the night and encourage the couple to maintain their joint interests and activities. If there are serious problems, marital therapy might be necessary. If Sue does have a depressive illness then treatment will be necessary, and there may be corresponding benefits in her relationship with her husband and child, but it is important to help the family recognise and deal with its own problems so that the family can move forward together.

CASE HISTORY 3

Mrs Ham brought her 11-year-old son, Jordan, into the practice. The doctor knew from his records that Jordan was an only child and that his parents had divorced a few years previously. In the surgery, Jordan sat sullenly in a chair with his arms folded, avoiding eye contact. 'There must be something wrong with him, doctor, he's never well enough to go to school.' Jordan had not been into school for a year despite the best efforts of Mrs Ham and an educational welfare officer. 'I sometimes get him as far as the school gates and he turns white and says that he feels shaky and unwell so he comes home and I ask him whether he'll try going in the next day, but he never goes past those gates. During the day he just lies in bed at home or plays computer games.'

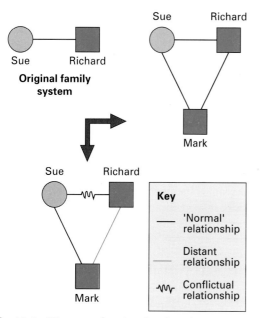

Fig. 10.1 Diagrams showing the changing relationships in Case history 2.

Key
— 'Normal' relationship
— Distant relationship
⁓⁓ Conflictual relationship

Is Jordan a truant?

No, because he does not absent himself from school to go off with friends or on his own to places that the school and his parent do not know about. He stays at home with his mother. His problems is one of *school refusal* not truancy.

Should doctors be concerned about school refusal?

On the surface the problem may appear to be more the province of the educational welfare officer or educational psychologist, but the family doctor has a vital role to play. The family doctor can help exclude physical illness (Jordan often says he is unwell before coming home) and also explore whether there are other health factors at play. A family doctor might want to exclude solvent or substance abuse. The psychological factors at play are also unclear. Perhaps Jordan is being bullied at school. Bullying causes a great deal of emotional distress to its victims and has been linked with suicide attempts. If he is being bullied he may have a depressive illness as a consequence.

The doctor may also want to explore the psychological rewards that *reinforce* and hence maintain Jordan's behaviour. The staying at home may reduce his anxiety and be *the primary reward*, but there may be *secondary rewards* such as his mother's attention and kindness, special food and computer games. A more covert reward may be his mother's approval. You might notice that when she describes how she tries to get him into school she says that she asks *him* whether or not he will go in the next day. It is clear that she yields her authority in this matter to him.

Mrs Ham says that she wants Jordan to go to school, so how might she also want Jordan at home?

Deep down Mrs Ham may prefer Jordan at home. He might provide her with someone to talk to, and she may be afraid that he will grow away from her and leave her as her husband did. Although she acknowledges his need to be educated, she may also like him being at home with her and so she may be half-hearted in her attempts to get him into school. She may be content to have tried and failed. Her bringing Jordan to the doctor may, in fact, have been the welfare officer's idea, not hers. She might not wholly want the doctor to succeed. If the doctor succeeded she would have to lose her son's com-

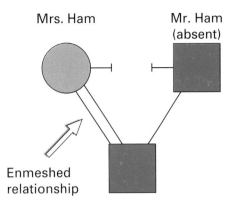

Fig. 10.2 The enmeshed relationship discussed in Case history 3.

pany. Thus she is rewarded by his company and he is rewarded by her tacit approval. They may have a relationship which is known as *enmeshed* because of its very close nature (see Fig. 10.2).

What can be done?

The situation is unfortunate because Jordan is losing contact with his peer group and not gaining the skills that will help him develop satisfying relationships later in life. He is losing out on his education and may never fulfil his potential in terms of any career. So, the stakes are very high, but any helping agency would have to acknowledge that they may be working against the family system. If both Mrs Ham and Jordan want him at home, then there is going to be little motivation for either of them to change. One or both of them need to accept the need for change and want to work towards it. Explaining the situation might help, although the arguments are probably very familiar to everyone concerned. Some work might be directed at reducing Jordan's anxieties about school. The educational psychologist and his teachers might work together so that he could be gradually reintroduced to the school a bit at a time as in a *systematic desensitisation* programme. Jordan might be encouraged to ventilate his feelings about his absent father either as an individual or in family therapy, and may even be treated for any low mood that might be present. Family work may encourage Mrs Ham to change the language she uses with Jordan. For instance, instead of *asking* Jordan she might start *telling* him to go into school. Even so, if mother and son lack sufficient motivation to make things work it may be necessary for other authorities to invoke legal proceedings that require parents to send their children to school. The legal dimension may show how seriously the problem is viewed by those in authority and may spur Mrs Ham to summon enough courage and authority herself to send Jordan to school.

CASE HISTORY 4

The concerned parents of William, 8, brought him along to see the child psychiatrist. William was less than 60% of the normal body mass for his height. When he could exercise he would exercise as hard as he could, although recently he had become too tired to run cross country, a sport which he had several junior medals for. For breakfast he would consume only hot water; for lunch dry bread and an orange; for supper an egg and an orange. His family doctor had put him on a weight chart, but William had cheated by drinking extra water on the days he was to be weighed.

When the psychiatrist interviewed him on his own William cried a lot. He seemed preoccupied with the death of his grandfather the previous year and also was worried that his father was spending weeks away from home. He said that he was worried about his father dying in a car crash. From the family interview it transpired that his father, a musician, played in a touring band which spent much time away from home. William's mother argued with his father about this during the family interview and indicated that this was a source of friction in the marriage. The mother also revealed that she had had anorexia nervosa when she was a teenager. Although she was no longer anorexic she confessed to being a 'fitness freak'.

What are the main problems outlined above?

William has made and is making strenuous efforts to lose weight and has succeeded in reducing his weight to levels that would fulfil the criteria for anorexia nervosa. Anorexia nervosa does occur in boys, but it is very uncommon. About 90% of anorexics are female.

His mood is very low following a bereavement and he shows much concern about his parents' marriage.

Besides anorexia nervosa what other diagnosis might be made?

William may have a depressive illness. His concerns about his grandfather's death and his parent's marriage sound all-consuming. The doctor would be interested in assessing the depth of his depression and its associated symptoms and signs. Although suicide is rare in children so young, it may be that William feels that life is not worth living and this would be an indicator of how severe his depression is. This would be one of the factors that determined whether or not William was admitted to hospital or treated in the community. His doctor could arrange some grief counselling or individual psychotherapy to help assess his mood, ease William's grief and tackle eating issues. Cognitive behavioural therapy may be used to treat the anorexia nervosa whether or not William is an in-patient or an out-patient. Antidepressants may be another option especially if it is felt that part of William's refusal to maintain his body weight is due to depressive appetite loss. Some tricyclic antidepressants often increase appetite as a side-effect besides elevating depressed mood. Child psychiatrists are often more reluctant to prescribe drugs than their adult counterparts, however, and more willing to consider individual, group and family therapies.

Family issues sound particularly important in this case. William's mother sounds as if she had anorexia nervosa herself, and there may be dysfunctional attitudes to food and fitness in the family. The whole family may be perfectionistic and put an overvalued premium on thinness and exercise. William may be struggling to succeed according to his parents' demanding criteria. A further family assessment by a family therapy team would be very helpful to try and defuse any direct or indirect criticism that exists within the family and to explore the family's ideas about eating, living together or apart and the role of (living or dead) grandparents. It might be useful to reassure William that, to some extent, the affairs of his parents (*the parental subsystem*) are not his to try and control and, conversely, communicate to his parents that they should maintain the boundaries of that subsystem (i.e. not allow worry to spill over unnecessarily into their offspring (*the children's subsystem*).

LEARNING POINTS

Child and adolescent psychiatry

- Boys are more prone to conduct disorders, girls are more prone to emotional disorders.
- Depression, especially in adolescent males, is becoming more frequent in older children.
- Family and marital problems often manifest as child psychiatric problems so family dynamics must be assessed before assuming that the pathology rests with the child alone.
- Childhood schizophrenia is exceedingly rare.
- Solvent and substance abuse is becoming more common in the young and may precipitate brief psychotic episodes.
- Child suicide is exceedingly rare, but is becoming more likely.

Self-assessment

MCQS

1 First-line treatments for childhood depression include:
   a tricyclic antidepressants
   b electroconvulsive therapy
   c individual psychotherapy
   d family therapy
   e group therapy

2 Which of the following statements are true or false?
   a Girls (aged less than 11) whose mothers die are at risk of becoming depressed as adults.
   b Children aged 5–10 years with emotional disorders are at greatly increased risk of psychiatric disorders as adults.
   c Many adults with schizoprehnia showed signs of neurodevelopmental immaturity as children.
   d Adults with bipolar affective disorder frequently had emotional disorders as a child.
   e Children with conduct disorders usually become adults with dissocial personality disorder.

Short answer questions

Write short notes on:
1 The emotional reactions of children to change in family structures.
2 The differences between conduct and emotional disorders.
3 Behavioural therapy in childhood psychological disorders.

MCQ answers

1 a = F,   b = F,   c = T,   d = T,   e = T
2 a = T,   b = F,   c = T,   d = F,   e = F

Explorations

Sources listed in the 'Further reading and reference' section will help you with the following.

Links with public health

What are the most common childhood mental disorders? What are the most common adolescent mental disorders? What is the ratio between boys and girls in these disorders? How can prevalence figures be obtained about childhood mental disorders?

Links with primary care

What proportion of children presenting to family doctors with abdominal pain have known physical diagnoses that account for the pain? How can GPs know when a child's abdominal pain is physical and when the pain is more to do with psychological or social factors? What might these non-physical factors be? How can the family doctor manage such a case?

Further reading and references

ADAMS P L 1973 Obsessive children. Penguin Books, New York

ADAMS S 1991 Prescribing of psychotropic drugs to children and adolescents. British Medical Journal 302: 217

BARKER P 1992 Basic family therapy, 3rd edn. Blackwell

BESAG V 1989 Bullies and victims in schools. Open University Press, Milton Keynes

Bowman F M, Garralda M E 1993 Psychiatric morbidity among children who are frequent attenders in general practice. British Journal of General Practice 43: 6–9

Cox A D 1988 Maternal depression and its impact on children's development. Archives of Disease in Childhood 63: 90–95

Garralda M E, Bailey D 1987 Psychosomatic aspects of children's consultations in primary care. European archives of psychiatry and neurological sciences 236: 319–322

Garralda M E, Bailey D 1989 Psychiatric disorders in general paediatric referrals. Archives of Disease in Childhood 64: 1727–1733

Hoare P 1993 Essential child psychiatry. Churchill Livingstone, Edinburgh

Leonard H L et al 1993 A two- to seven-year follow-up study of 54 obsessive compulsive children and adolescents. Archives of General Psychiatry 149: 1244–1251

Murray L, Cooper P J, Stein A 1991 Postnatal depression and infant development. British Medical Journal 302: 978–979

Russell G, Szmukler G, Dare C, Eisler I 1987 An evaluation of family therapy in anorexia nervosa and bulimia nervosa. Archives of General Psychiatry 44: 1047–1057

Rutter M, Taylor E, Hersov L 1994 Child and adolescent psychiatry: modern approaches, 3rd edn. Blackwell Scientific Publications, Oxford

11

Sexual aspects of psychiatry

Human sexuality is a vital and integral part of behaviour and personality. Sexual dysfunction is a source of great distress to individuals and couples. Sexual dysfunction may lead to a failure to form relationships or the breakup of existing relationships and families.

Contents

Male sexual problems

Problems of desire

The sexual drive or libido is inherent in all human beings. Usually the sexual drive is directed towards appropriate sexual partners, but sometimes there can be problems with the drive in terms of its amount or direction. Loss of libido implies a diminution in the sexual drive and can be caused by psychological disorders such as depression and anorexia nervosa and physical illnesses such as carcinomatosis or heart failure. Excess libido can be associated with psychological disorders such as hypomania or frontal lobe syndrome or rarely physical illnesses such as tuberculosis.

The libido may be directed unconventionally, as in homosexuality. Homosexuality among both men and women was once, but is no longer, classed as a psychiatric disorder. Less socially acceptable objects of desire include children (*paedophilia*) and animals (*bestiality*). Arousal may also be associated with objects (*fetishism*), such as high-heeled shoes and leather, or be associated with inflicting pain (*sadism*) or having pain inflicted upon one (*masochism*). *Transvestism* is a behaviour where arousal is produced by dressing in clothes appropriate to the opposite sex (*cross-dressing*). Transvestites may be heterosexually or homosexually oriented.

Problems of gender

Apart from biological intersex conditions, gender is generally appropriately assigned by society according to the normal male's genitalia. The social gender given to the new-born male is usually followed by a core male gender. In other words, the male looks and feels that he is a male. In *male transsexuals*, although male genitalia are fully developed, the core gender is female. So although phenotypically male, the *male transsexual* feels that he is female and should have female genitalia. There is a fundamental difference from male homosexuals who both look male and feel that they are males. Male transsexuals may cross-dress and seek hormonal and surgical means of adopting feminine attributes.

Problems of performance

Because of social taboos, the sexual act is shrouded in a certain aura of mystery. The sexually naive individual or couple may lack the necessary knowledge and skills to perform sex. Doctors do not help this process: they often overestimate their patient's knowledge of sexual anatomy and function and often fail to explain sexual matters clearly.

Lacking the confidence that experience can bring, a young man may suffer with *premature ejaculation*, where semen is ejaculated before entering the vagina, or before sex has properly got underway. The problem may lead to avoidance of the sexual act (a bit like the avoidance associated with a phobia) and problems in relationships.

CASE HISTORY 1

Simon came to his family doctor twice before he said what he wanted to say. The first time he spoke to the female partner in the general practice and came away red-faced, clutching a prescription for a sore throat. The second time Simon attended he saw a young male doctor who spent some time trying to understand Simon's anxiety. Simon told him that he was having problems with his girlfriend and that she had told him to 'get it sorted out, because there must be something wrong with you'. Amidst some embarrassment the teenager told the doctor that when he tried to have sex with his girlfriend 'it didn't last very long'. On careful questioning about what Simon meant, it transpired that Simon always ejaculated during foreplay. He had never managed to penetrate his partner. The closest that they had both got to intercourse was when he managed to put a condom on. Unfortunately, he ejaculated immediately afterwards.

What can the doctor do to help?

Talking about the problem in a straightforward way will help defuse some of the anxiety that Simon feels. People are often greatly troubled by sexual problems, but wonder whether their doctor can help, or will even be prepared to listen. In this case the doctor is careful to find out exactly what Simon means when he says 'it didn't last very long' — doctors are used to taking long histories about pains and other presenting complaints, but are all too often prepared to take statements about sexual problems at face value.

Feeding back what the doctor understands the problem to be (i.e. premature ejaculation) will enable Simon to correct any misapprehensions on the doctor's part and will begin to help explain matters. Education about sex using explanations, diagrams, videos or books may help as may further practice. Engaging both partners in helping each other with the problem often reduces anxiety, improves the relationship and allows other issues to be discussed between the couple. Giving permission for the couple to experiment may defuse tension. The female partner may be asked to help the male ejaculate outside the vagina, and they may work together in prolonging the sexual encounter by stimulating so far then stopping before male orgasm (*stop-start technique*). Once control is established in this way, the couple might progress to vaginal penetration. Such simple psychological management is often all that is required, but the doctor needs to follow the case up. Individuals may go away from the doctor and the doctor may wrongly assume that the problem is solved when they do not return. People may be too embarrassed to return, so the doctor needs to make things easier for them to do so by making a further appointment.

What if the problem does not get better?

Some simple physical techniques can be used by the couple, such as the *squeeze technique* (Fig. 11.1) in addition to the stop-start technique. A behavioural programme which relies on *sensate focus* could be used, as in Table 11.1. In the sensate focus technique the doctor prescribes a total cessation of attempts at sexual intercourse and, instead, introduces a series of graded tasks. These graded tasks slowly lead from simple caressing to full penetration. The effect of initially prohibiting intercourse enhances this as a goal, but also reduces anxiety associated with performance. Couples can focus on simple ways of giving each other pleasure that do not rely upon penetration.

There may be underlying problems in the relationship that need to be resolved and relationship

---

Table 11.1 An example of a sensate focus programme

1 Therapist asks couple to take it in turns to touch each other's body, when in private, comfortable and unclothed. Therapists forbids couple to have sexual intercourse or touch each other's genitals.
2 Partners tell each other only if some touching is unpleasant. The touching is then changed.
3 In the next stage the couple is asked to touch each other and say what they like as well as saying what they find uncomfortable.
4 Problems with 'assignment' are discussed.
5 Genital touching is allowed and stages 2 and 3 are repeated. The 'stop-start' technique is incorporated. Orgasm is allowed, but is not the prime aim of touching. Communication is stressed.
6 Subsequent stages involve brief vaginal entry, or different positions, leading to sexual intercourse.

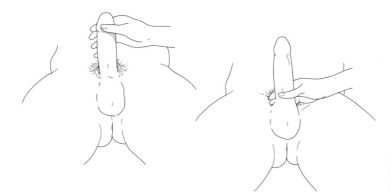

Fig. 11.1 Squeeze technique. Pressure under the corona or on the bottom of the penis can delay ejaculation.

counselling as provided by organisations such as Relate may be helpful.

Pharmacological means of retarding ejaculation can be tried. Fluoxetine, as a side-effect, can delay ejaculation, and a short course of the drug may be sufficient to restore confidence.

Male *impotence* is either a complete failure to attain an erection or an inability to maintain an erection. Classically the problem is seen in older men, but can affect all ages. When the erection commonly occurring on waking is also absent, thought must be given to an underlying organic cause (such as diabetes mellitus or alcoholism). Anxiety is a common psychological cause of impotence. Often a mixture of physical and psychological factors may interact to produce impotence (Table 11.2).

CASE HISTORY 2

Graham, 24, attended his family doctor after his wife left him. He had only been married for 2 months. His initial complaint was that he was not sleeping. He asked for some sleeping tablets. His doctor, who did not know about the separation, asked him about his wife because she knew that he had only just got married. Graham became tearful and said that he had been responsible for his wife's leaving. He was reluctant to say why,

but eventually admitted that they had been unable to consummate the marriage. Despite his wanting to have sex and his enjoyment of foreplay to a limited extent, he felt somehow threatened by the idea of entering his wife. He was, he said, frightened of what would happen. His wife had been understanding at first, but had grown angry with him. Now he was even more afraid. With tactful questioning the doctor elicited some important facts from his psychosexual history. Graham had never had a girlfriend before his wife and they had never attempted sex before marriage. Graham also disclosed (for the first time in his life to anyone) that he had been sexually abused by an uncle when he was 10. He had deep feelings of regret about this and the whole area of sexual behaviour was clouded by the feeling that it was dirty and forbidden.

What can the doctor do to investigate a diagnosis?

There are strong pointers to a psychological cause for Graham's impotence — his avoidance of sex in the past, his fear of penetrating his wife and continuing feelings about childhood sexual abuse (which he has been unable to disclose to his wife). The doctor needs to ask more questions about Graham's normal sexual functioning — is he able to get an erection in other circumstances? Can he masturbate to orgasm? These questions are not intended to pry, but to establish whether Graham has the ability to function physiologically (see Table 11.2 for organic causes of erectile dysfunction). The hypothesis would then be that psychological factors are inhibiting normal physiological functioning.

If the doctor suspects that organic factors may be playing a part in the impotence (although there are no particular features in the case above) a variety of investigations are open to her. The majority of cases of impotence have physical causes and a physical examination followed by simple screening blood tests may alert the family doctor to problems. Suitable first-line investigations may be a full blood count, serum urea and electrolytes, thyroid function tests (if indicated) and serum testosterone.

Graham has found it possible to confide in his

Table 11.2   Physical causes of male impotence

Illness and disease
- Alcoholism (neuropathy)
- Diabetes mellitus
- Arterial disease, e.g. Leriche syndrome
- Renal failure
- Carcinomatosis
- Neurosyphilis
- Hypothalamo-pituitary dysfunction
- Liver failure
- Multiple sclerosis and many others

Drugs
- Beta-blockers
- Thiazide diuretics
- Tricyclic antidepressants
- Phenothiazines
- Spironolactone
- Cimetidine
- Cannabis
- Antiepileptics

family doctor and the relationship is probably, therefore, an important one to him. If the family doctor can manage the case herself, then this might be useful — the management would consist of excluding organic causes and counselling Graham about sexual function and exploring his feelings about the past abuse. The family doctor may not wish to undertake this counselling or therapy herself, but refer Graham to a psychiatrist who specialises in psychosexual medicine or an experienced counsellor.

Physical treatments are available which can promote erections. Once the erection is attained sexual intercourse can occur. Successful intercourse hopefully leads to increased confidence and a short course of such treatments can break the cycle of low self-esteem and performance anxiety. The physical treatment involves intrapenile injections of papaverine or prostaglandin E_1 given into the corpora cavernosum. Cases of neurogenic impotence and psychogenic impotence respond with erection, but where arterial insufficiency is a problem erection may be impossible even with intra-cavernosal injections. External vacuum devices can help produce erections and are sometimes seen as more acceptable than self-administered injections.

LEARNING POINTS

Male sexual problems

- The most common male sexual problems that present to specialist clinics are impotence (or erectile failure) and premature ejaculation.
- Psychogenic impotence is a diagnosis of exclusion. Physical causes account for the majority of cases, underlining the importance of medical training and diagnostic skills.
- Where organic causes of sexual dysfunction have been excluded, management consists of improving the individual's and couple's knowledge about sex, enhancing their communication skills and teaching simple behavioural techniques to use during sex.
- Intensive psychotherapy is reserved for patients where internal conflicts about gender identity can be identified or where there are repeated patterns of relationship behaviours that can be changed.

- Erections can be produced by the intracavernosal injection of papaverine or prostaglandin E_1 or the use of external vacuum devices.

Female sexual problems

Problems of desire

The most common female sexual problem presenting to specialist clinics is one of low sexual interest. This problem is relatively difficult to treat. It may require intensive psychotherapy looking at reasons for an ambivalence about sexual behaviour caused, say, by childhood sexual abuse. Organic causes such as endocrine disturbance (hypothyroidism, hyperthyroidism, Cushing's disease, pituitary adenomas and others) need to be excluded as do psychiatric disorders like depression. Hysterectomy and mastectomy seriously affect self-image and appropriate counselling may help patients overcome difficulties in resuming sexual behaviour after such operations. Hysterectomy and mastectomy patients often need to mourn the loss of their uterus or breast. Their partners often need to be involved, although commonly resist inclusion and 'deny' problems. Fear of recurrent disease does not help matters. Appropriate exploration of fears and reasonable reassurance may help, but a depressive reaction and treatment for this must be considered.

Problems of gender

Transsexualism occurs in women, but is probably about three times less common than in men. Transsexual behaviour can manifest as early as middle childhood. There is no good current evidence of a genetic mechanism, but some studies suggest that some female to male transsexuals may have raised testosterone levels and a higher incidence of polycystic ovarian disease. Even so, environmental and cultural factors are thought to be more important than biological factors.

Problems of performance

Dyspareunia is pain felt during sexual intercourse. Although dyspareunia can occur in men, it is 10 times more common in women. Organic causes such as vaginal infection or irritation and post-menopausal dryness and atrophic vaginitis are common and must either be treated or excluded before too much reliance is placed on a purely psychological hypothesis. Table 11.3 shows some causes of dyspareunia. Despite this it must be recognised that even where there are organic causes of dyspareunia, psychological factors may have a part to play. For instance, difficulties in the relationship may lead to inadequate foreplay resulting in inadequate vaginal lubrication before penetration causing discomfort during and after intercourse and a resulting cycle of anger and disharmony in the couple. Alternatively, the memory of past sexual trauma or damage done during childbirth may account for a change in the perception of the experience.

Similar ambivalent feelings about sex in general, or the partner in particular, may lead to *vaginismus*, an inability to allow penetration of the vagina associated with spasm of the perineal muscles, *sexual aversion*, *lack of enjoyment*, and *anorgasmia* (the lack of orgasm).

CASE HISTORY 3

A teenager called Clare was referred to a female gynaecologist because she had pain when her boyfriend tried to make love to her. She had refused to let her male family doctor examine her then, just as she had refused to allow him to examine her when she had requested the contraceptive pill a few months before. The family doctor had felt unable to issue a prescription for the pill and the relationship between him and Clare was strained.

The gynaecologist took a careful and sensitive history from Clare. It transpired that she had never been able to allow any of her boyfriends to enter or even touch her vagina. She was sure that her vagina was too small and would burst if she allowed anything inside it. When her boyfriend put on a condom and tried to enter her she 'froze rigid' and all her muscles went tense.

What can the gynaecologist do?

She can assess what knowledge Clare has about female anatomy and what her sex education was like. What beliefs or fears does she have about the size of her vagina? What are Clare's feelings about sex? Is she very worried about becoming pregnant without the contraceptive pill? Her anxieties are probably contributing to an increased pelvic muscle tone which would make entry painful or impossible (vaginismus), therefore reinforcing the idea that she cannot accommodate an erect penis. Simple education and a gradual and gentle vaginal examination by the gynaecologist, (perhaps using Clare's own fingers first) may change some of Clare's ideas about her own body and be all that is required. Sometimes the use of graded dilators by the patient and then her partner may help.

Table 11.3 Physical causes of dyspareunia

Female
- Failure of vaginal lubrication
- Failure of vasocongestion
- Failure of uterine elevation and vaginal ballooning during arousal
- Oestrogen deficiency leading to atrophic vaginitis
- Radiotherapy for malignancy
- Vaginal infection, e.g. *Trichomonas* or herpes
- Vaginal irritation, e.g. sensitivity to creams or deodorants
- Abnormal tone of pelvic floor muscles
- Scarring after episiotomy or surgery
- Bartholin's gland cysts/abscess
- Rigid hymen, small introitus

Male
- Painful retraction of the foreskin
- Herpetic and other infections
- Asymmetrical erection due to fibrosis or Peyronie's disease
- Hypersensitivity of the glans penis

LEARNING POINTS

Female sexual problems

- The most common female sexual problem seen in specialist clinics is one of low sexual interest, which may have physical and psychological causes.
- Most non-organic problems can be relieved by open discussion, education and involvement of the partner.
- Doctors should also seek to improve communication between the partners so that each part-

ner's desires and needs begin to be clearly expressed and listened to.

- Underlying psychiatric disorders, such as depression, require treatment.

Self-assessment

MCQs

1 Common sexual problems include:
   a transsexualism
   b erectile dysfunction
   c male dyspareunia
   d premature ejaculation
   e vaginismus

2 Causes of a reduction in libido or erectile dysfunction include:
   a antihypertensive drugs
   b haemochromatosis
   c diabetes mellitus
   d hypothyroidism
   e hyperthyroidism

3 Useful treatments for:
   a erectile dysfunction include intrapenile injections of paroxetine
   b premature ejaculation include the squeeze technique
   c homosexuality include aversion therapy
   d vaginismus include the 'stop-start' technique
   e premature ejaculation include fluoxetine

MCQ answers

1 a = F, b = T, c = F, d = T, e = F
2 All true
3 a = F, b = T, c = F, d = F, e = T

Explorations

Links with genetics, embryology and anatomy

How do problems with male and female genotypes express themselves phenotypically? What causes do you know for intersex states? What psychological reactions might occur in children with anatomically abnormal sexual organs?

Links with physiology

How is sexual function linked in to the female reproductive cycle? How is the reproductive cycle controlled? How might psychological stress interfere with gonadotrophin production?

What sensory inputs lead to male arousal? How can cortical activity modulate arousal? What changes in penile blood flow lead to erection? How can damage to pelvic nerves affect this process?

Links with communication skills

How might patients with sexual problems present to their family doctor? What communication skills of the doctor will enable him or her to pick up these problems? What kind of language should be used in exploring sexual problems and explaining proposed management of these problems?

Links with gynaecology

How common is dyspareunia? What is the age distribution of women presenting with the problem? What effect does age have on sexual function?

Further reading and references

BANCROFT J 1989 Human sexuality and its problems, 2nd edn. Churchill Livingstone, Edinburgh

CRANSTON-CUEBAS M A, BARLOW D H 1990 Cognitive and affective contributions to sexual functioning. Annual Review of Sex Research 1: 119–162

GREEN R 1985 Gender identity in childhood and later sexual orientation: follow-up of 78 males. American Journal of Psychiatry 142: 339–341

KINSEY A C, POMEROY W B, MARTIN C E 1948 Sexual behaviour in the human male. Saunders, Philadelphia

KINSEY A C, POMEROY W B, MARTIN C E, GEBHARD P H 1953 Sexual behaviour in the human female. Saunders, Philadelphia

LIPSIUS S H 1987 Prescribing sensate focus without proscribing intercourse. Journal of Sexual and Marital Therapy 13(2): 106–16

MASTERS W H, JOHNSON V E 1970 Human sexual inadequacy. Churchill, London

MATHERS N et al 1994 Assessment of training in psychosexual medicine. British Medical Journal 308: 969–972

POLLACK M H, REITER S, HAMMERNESS P 1992 Genitourinary and sexual adverse effects of psychotropic medication. International Journal of Psychiatry and Medicine 22(4): 305–27

WALBROEHL G S 1987 Sexuality in the handicapped. American Family Physician 36(1): 129–33

WYATT G E, PETERS S D, GUTHRIE D 1988 Kinsey revisited, Part I: Comparisons of the sexual socialization and sexual behavior of white women over 33 years. Archives of Sexual Behaviour 17(3): 201–39

Sexual problems in literature

Burgess A Earthly Powers
Nabokov V Lolita
Amis K The Old Devils
Davies P The Rebel Angels

—— **Resources** ——————

Institute of Psychosexual Medicine,
11 Chandos Street,
Cavendish Square,
London W1M 9DE
Tel: 0171 580 0631

Relate,
Herbert Gray College,
Little Church,
Rugby CV21 13AP.
(Look in telephone directory for local address/telephone number)

Psychiatry and old age

Although elderly people generally enjoy relatively good health, the ageing brain is more susceptible to physical insults than the brain of a younger adult. Various pathological processes such as cerebrovascular disease and amyloid plaque formation may cause a global deterioration in brain function called dementia. The elderly with normal cognitive functions are susceptible to a range of mental disorders that affect younger adults too. Affected by bereavements, loneliness and failing health some elderly people may suffer with depressive illness.

Contents

The ageing brain

The brain of a 75 year old has been subjected to a lifetime of brain insults which may have included events such as birth injuries, head trauma, viral infections, episodes of hypoxia, exposure to environmental toxins such as lead and transient ischaemic attacks amongst others. This catalogue of events, together with normal ageing processes in the brain, means that the functional reserves of the aged brain are diminished compared to a healthy 25 year old. This fall in the 'cerebral reserve' is diagrammatically represented in Figure 12.1.

Memory function in elderly persons is less good, partially because of reduced learning ability for new information. Although memories of long ago may still be as bright, the ageing brain is functionally less plastic and new memories are less easily formed. This is usually a relatively benign memory impairment.

Because the cerebral reserve has been diminished, further brain insults, such as an episode of chest infection, may not be coped with. A similar infection in a 25 year old with higher cerebral reserves may pass without any observable deterioration in brain function. In a 75 year old, however, the infection may so use up the reserve capacity that confusion supervenes. In other words, the ageing brain is increasingly vulnerable to new insults and, if burdened, easily descends into a transient confusional state.

The prevalence of mental disorders in the elderly

Dementia from all causes may be present in about 4–5% of the population over the age of 65. Over the age of 85 the prevalence rises to about 20%. Depression requiring treatment may be present in about 10% of the population over 65. Most cases of depression in the elderly go unrecognised and untreated.

Dementia

Dementia is a chronic and progressive global deterioration of brain function. The causes of dementia are varied, although Alzheimer-type dementia is one of the commonest (see Table 12.1). Some of the causes are partially or wholly reversible with treatment, like hypothyroidism or Wilson's disease, so accurate diagnosis is very important.

Unlike acute organic brain syndrome (delirium), the onset of dementia is often gradual and its progress slow. In senile dementia of the Alzheimer type (SDAT) the course of the illness from first symptoms/signs to death may be 6 years or more.

The symptoms and signs of dementia reflect the parts of the brain which are damaged by the disease process, so that difficulties with the task of dressing or the order of tasks in dressing may reflect cortical damage in the parietal lobe. Some dementias affect cortical *and* subcortical structures. Others, like

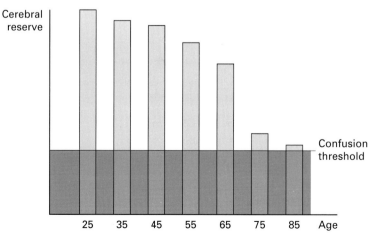

Fig. 12.1 'Cerebral reserve' decreases with age. A brain insult that a 25-year-old brain could function in spite of may well push and submerge a 75-year-old brain below the confusion threshold

Table 12.1   Causes of dementia

- Alzheimer's disease
- Lewy body disease
- Multi-infarct dementia (arteriosclerotic dementia)
- Alcoholic dementia
- Binswanger's disease
- Creutzfeldt-Jakob disease
- Huntington's chorea
- AIDS related dementia
- Parkinson's disease
- Normal pressure hydrocephalus
- Other genetic causes, e.g. Wilson's disease
- Metabolic disease, e.g. hypothyroidism
- Malnutrition, e.g. vitamin deficiencies
- Toxic or traumatic injury, e.g. carbon monoxide poisoning or traumatic brain damage
- Malignant disease; primary or metastatic
- Infections, e.g. neurosyphilis

Table 12.2   Some clinical features in cortical dementia syndromes

- Short-term memory impairment (anterograde amnesia)
  — Forgetting appointments
  — Losing personal possessions, e.g. glasses
  — Self-neglect — forgetting to wash, forgetting meals
- Long-term memory impairment
  — Late feature
- Agnosias
  — e.g. Visual agnosia
  — Topographical agnosia (getting lost)
  — Hemisomatoagnosia
- Dyspraxias, e.g.
  — Constructional
  — Dressing
- Dysphasias, e.g.
  — Expressive
  — Receptive
  — Nominal
- Dyscalculia
- Difficulty remembering names or recognising others (or even self in mirror)
- Disinhibition and poor judgement, risk of being exploited
- Perseveration, echolalia, palilalia, echopraxias
- Disorientation in time, place and person
- Incontinence
- Return of primitive reflexes
- Emotional lability: tearfulness or anger
- Depression
- Mistaken beliefs
  — e.g. that parents are still alive or that children are still at school

Binswanger's disease, tend to affect just the subcortical structures and therefore have different symptom profiles. A key early clinical feature of most dementias, however, is short-term memory loss, which is really an inability to form new memories (anterograde amnesia). Long-term memories may be intact, although later in the illness these too may be lost, so that patients may fail to remember their marriages or fail to recognise their spouses.

Carers may also have to cope with changes in the patient's personality. From earlier chapters you will have learnt how lesions in the frontal lobe can affect personality by removing inhibitions. For example, dementia patients with lesions in their frontal lobe may swear (where they never have done before), insult others or make inappropriate sexual advances to strangers. Frontal lesions are also associated with a loss of continence. Dementia patients may occasionally be violent where this has never been a feature of their personality before. Psychotic symptoms such as visual hallucinations may also occur. Not every patient with a dementia has exactly the same symptoms or follows the same course. Table 12.2 gives a list of possible dementia symptoms and signs. Table 12.3 shows some key features of different dementias.

CASE HISTORY 1

Mary had been married for 42 years when her husband Fred died of lung cancer. She found coping with the arrangements after his death very difficult and leaned heavily on her friends and relatives. This they could understand, but weeks after the funeral, Mary still seemed very disorganised. Friends would call round to the house and find it in a mess, with half-empty milk bottles and partly finished meals in odd places about the house. When they made arrangements to see her Mary would not keep the appointments. When they mentioned these missed appointments to Mary she would become upset.

Her brother-in-law first noticed there was something seriously wrong when Mary phoned asking him where he was, claiming that he had forgotten to come and pick her up to take her to work. For one thing Mary had retired some years

Table 12.3 Distinguishing features of some dementias

Dementia	Onset	Brain pathology	Transmission	Key clinical features
SDAT	Early form 50+ Late form 65+	Cortical thinning and ventricular dilatation Senile plaques and neurofibrillary tangles	Early onset form possibly autosomal dominant Late onset form four times more likely in first degree relatives	Anterograde amnesia and cortical dementia features (see Table 12.2)
Multi-infarct	65+	Focal infarcts in white matter showing as areas of low attenuation on CT/MRI scans		Stepwise, deterioration Onset sometimes sudden Focal neurological signs
Huntington's	30–40 years	Abnormal GABA and dopamine systems in basal ganglia Reduced volume of caudate and putamen on CT/MRI	Autosomal dominant gene on chromosome 4	Involuntary movements, gait abnormalities
Parkinson's	65+	Subcortical dementia in 20% of Parkinson's		Associated with Parkinsonian features
Normal pressure hydrocephalus	Usually 60+	Dilatation of ventricles without cortical thinning on CT/MRI scans		Unexplained incontinence and gait abnormalities
Prion dementia (Creutzfeldt-Jakob disease)	Adulthood	Accumulated prion protein Astrocytosis Spongiform appearance No cerebral atrophy	Horizontal rather than vertical	Rapidly progressive dementia, most dead within 2 years Abnormal movements and EEG
AIDS	< 65	Brain atrophy Thickened meninges Demyelination Astrocytosis	Horizontal and vertical	Slow onset Tremor, ataxia, hyperreflexia, dysarthria Frontal release signs
Wilson's	< 65	Copper deposition in basal ganglia	Autosomal recessive	Kayser-Fleischer rings around iris Abnormal movements
Pick's	55–60	Frontal and temporal lobe atrophy Pick's bodies and ballon cells	Incomplete penetrance of autosomal dominant gene	Personality change and euphoric mood
Neurosyphilis (general paralysis of the insane)	5–25 years after infection	Neuronal cell loss Astrocytosis *Treponema pallidum* in cortex	Horizontal and vertical	Small, unequal, unreactive pupils Disinhibition

ago, and for another it was 2 a.m. Two days later she turned up at their house in a taxi at 5 a.m. Her brother-in-law was so concerned that he took her to see her doctor.

What are the main problems identified by the friends and relatives?

These centre around Mary's disorganisation: she forgets appointments and seems to have lost her sense of time, doing daytime things when she should be asleep. Her mistake about whether or not she is working suggests a serious disorientation.

Why has this problem presented now?

The answer to this question depends upon the diagnosis. Mary is presenting after her husbands's death. It is possible that her bereavement reaction is so bad that she has become severely depressed. In older people depression can seem to change their cognitive abilities so much that they appear demented. This is called a pseudodementia, and it tends to resolve after the depression is appropriately treated. This could explain the time relationship between the death and her confused presentation.

On the other hand, the problem as related above does not highlight low mood as a prime feature, and there may be an alternative explanation for the presentation after Fred's death. Mary may have been becoming more disorientated and more disorganised for some time before his death and he may have been compensating for her. He may have been tidying away after her, and making sure that she did not miss her appointments, for instance. Sometimes a couple can be so symbiotic that the outside observer may not pick up the dementia symptoms in one of the partners at all. For instance, people with dementia sometimes have difficulty in remembering names or small details. If their partner is with them, he or she may prompt the other in such a natural way that any observer may think nothing of it. It is only when the partner is not present that the symptoms and signs of the dementia begin to be apparent.

How would you make the diagnosis?

A full history from the patient and an informant may yield important information such as a family history of early deaths from dementia or cerebrovascular disease. A past medical history of hypothyroidism, anaemia or stroke may be equally important. Look at the differential diagnosis of dementia (Table 12.3) and work out what features might be present in the history for each. Classically, senile dementia of the Alzheimer type (SDAT) follows a gradually deteriorating course, whereas a cerebrovascular dementia follows a stepwise deteriorating course with each sudden deterioration following a cerebrovascular event. This is information that can be gained from the history. Informants may be able to tell you how much the patient can do for themselves. Dressing apraxias can be detected in this way.

A physical examination is absolutely essential to pick up signs of Parkinsonism, say, or hypertension. Treatable causes of dementia, such as hypothyroidism, must be found and a physical examination might turn up features such as dry skin, hair loss, slow reflexes or bradycardia.

Physical investigations also need to be done: a full blood count (why?), serum B_{12} and folate, urea and electrolytes, thyroid function tests, liver function tests and syphilis screening would all be very relevant. If you find features in the history or physical examination which make you think of a specific disorder, more specialised tests may be warranted. If you found features of Wilson's disease, for example, what blood tests would you order? Radiological examinations such as chest X-rays and increasingly CT brain scans are routine initial assessments. An ECG is very important to exclude rhythm disturbances. Atrial fibrillation may, for example, predispose to embolus formation.

A mental state examination would elicit whether depressive symptoms are present. Specialised cognitive screening tests can be done here, e.g. looking for parietal lobe signs like dyscalculia or constructional dyspraxia which, if positive, would increase the likelihood of a dementing illness.

What can be done for dementia?

Dementias with treatable causes, such as hypothyroidism and Wilson's disease, may wholly or partially remit with treatment. Other dementias such as Alzheimer's and Huntington's are not yet treatable, although research is ongoing. Some treatments, such as *tacrine*, aim to enhance cholinergic neurotransmission in Alzheimer's dementia and have had limited results, but tacrine has serious side effects such as hepatotoxicity. The treatment of such patients is, therefore, care rather than cure; meeting their needs, prolonging their independence as long as possible and reducing the burden on carers as much as possible through the use of day hospitals, day centres and respite care are the aims in these cases.

CASE HISTORY 2

Edna, 78, did not go out of the house very often. It was a huge effort for her because she was plagued by osteoarthritis of the hips and was waiting for a hip replacement. Her home help did all her shopping and cleaning. Edna's closest friend had died in the summer and now, in October, she felt 'blue' as she described it. She struggled down to the family doctor one day to ask for sleeping tablets, as her joints were hurting more than usual. She said 'it was either that or a slug of whisky' although she had always been teetotal.

During the 5 minute conversation she had with her the family doctor noted how much weight Edna had lost. Although she knew that this would be good from the point of view of Edna's joints, she suspected that Edna had lost her appetite. When asked, Edna confirmed that food did not taste as good as it used to.

The family doctor acquiesced and gave Edna a short course of sleeping tablets, but arranged for the practice community psychiatric nurse (CPN) to call round to see her. He was able to spend much more time speaking to Edna about her loneliness and the loss of her lifelong friend. He also spoke to Edna's home help who said that lately Edna would sit silently in her chair for hours on end. The home help made her hot drinks, wrapped blankets about her and made sure the heating was on, but was worried in case the old lady developed hypothermia. When the home help knew Edna was not listening she told the CPN that Edna often 'shed a tear' nowadays.

What are the main problems here?

- Painful, osteoarthritic joints.
- Loneliness following bereavement.
- Risk of hypothermia.
- Insomnia.
- Low mood with tearfulness and psychomotor retardation.
- Poor appetite and weight loss.

The last three problems suggest that the patient has a depressive illness. It would be important to clarify the exact type of insomnia. Is the insomnia due to depression or physical causes? Is early morning wakening present? Is waking purely due to arthritic pain? If waking were the only problem and was purely due to pain then suitable analgesics might be more appropriate than an antidepressant. However, there are other features of depression, and depressive illness often interacts with pain to make pain seem much worse.

The weight loss as a symptom is perhaps less diagnostic of depression than in younger adults. It is important to realise that weight loss can indicate other illnesses such as heart failure, respiratory failure and malignant disease.

Is it worth treating depression if the causes seem mainly either physical or out of the doctor's control?

One of the reasons why older people may not receive the treatment they need for depression is the mistaken belief that if a depression is 'understandable' then it does not merit treatment. A doctor might say to himself 'Well, Edna is 78, she hasn't got much to look forward to. She is crippled with arthritis and her best friend died recently. I'd be depressed if I were her.' The important thing to remember is that depression is not normal in old age and that treatment is extremely worthwhile. Successful treatment for Edna would mean a better quality of life, might reduce her pain levels, increase her mobility and give her the confidence to go out and make new friends.

What treatments could be useful?

Most treatments available for younger adults are also suitable for the elderly, with some reservations.

Tricyclic antidepressants are cardiotoxic and an ECG would be important before starting therapy with these. Some tricyclics like doxepin and lofepramine are relatively less cardiotoxic. Electroconvulsive therapy is relatively safer than tricyclic medication and useful if psychotic symptoms are present. The anaesthetist may need to advise regarding the anaesthetic for electroconvulsive therapy. Many psychotropic drugs cause postural hypotension and this is a complication to be aware of since it may lead to falls and fractures. Newer antidepressants such as the SSRIs seem less prone to affect the heart or cause falls.

Cognitive behavioural therapy and bereavement counselling may be useful in the elderly. Day centres and day hospitals can be useful to combat loneliness and monitor recovery.

Other psychiatric disorders

First time presentations of hypomania and neurotic disorders are rare in the elderly and may signify some treatable organic pathology. Once treatable causes have been ruled out, symptomatic relief with conventional treatments in altered doses are useful. Schizophrenia does not tend to present in the elderly, but a variant, sometimes called paraphrenia, exists and is characterised by persecutory delusions and hallucinations. This disorder is more common in those who have sensory deficits, such as deafness, and the disorder's emergence may signify a dementing process.

LEARNING POINTS

Psychiatry and old age

- Ten per cent of the population over 65 has depressive illness. Despite this, most cases of depression in the elderly go unrecognised and untreated.
- Depression in the elderly is not normal and can be effectively treated.
- Depression can mimic dementia when attention and concentration are badly affected. This pseudodementia resolves with antidepressant therapy.
- Dementia affects about 5% of the elderly population.
- Some dementias are long illnesses (e.g. Alzheimer's, which lasts about 6 years from onset to death) while others are short (e.g. Creutzfeldt-Jakob, which lasts about 2 years).
- Symptoms and signs of dementia can help you localise lesions to specific areas in the grey and white matter.
- Most people with dementia are cared for at home by spouses or other relatives. These carers need practical and emotional support, but this support is usually underprovided.

Self-assessment

MCQs

1 Reversible causes of dementia include:
  a Pick's disease
  b Huntington's chorea
  c hypothyroidism
  d Creutzfeldt-Jakob disease
  e Wilson's disease

2 In a community of 2000 people over the age of 65:
  a about 200 would have dementia
  b about 200 might have depression
  c 300 would have obsessional-compulsive disorder
  d about 10 would have Huntington's chorea
  e at least 100 would have cerebrovascular dementia

3 Features of subcortical dementias include:
  a memory loss
  b dyscalculia
  c receptive aphasia
  d disorientation
  e tactile agnosia

MCQ answers

1 a = F, b = F, c = T, d = F, e = T
2 a = F, b = T, c = F, d = F, e = F
3 a = T, b = F, c = F, d = T, e = F

Explorations

Sources listed in the 'Further reading and reference' section will help you with the following.

Links with anatomy, physiology, pathology and neurology

Using the anatomy of the cerebral vasculature, find out which areas of the brain are mainly supplied by which arteries. Which of these arterial systems is most likely to become occluded? What therefore are the most likely brain areas to be damaged by strokes? How would these present to the doctor? What clinical signs might be elicited by the examining doctor, initially and after several days?

Links with sociology and psychology

What changes in their roles do older people face? How

do they and their families adapt to this changing role? How might the doctor or the health care team be called upon to help in this adjustment by the individual and family?

Links with public health medicine

What proportion of your local population is over 65? How are their mental health needs addressed in terms of *finding* morbidity and treatment once detected. Using prevalence and incidence statistics for depression and dementia in the elderly, estimate the actual number of cases in your local population. What services (local and central government run, voluntary and private) are available in your area? What changes are expected in the numbers of people in various age bands in your local population? What service changes are currently being planned to coincide with this change?

Links with histopathology

What are the histological changes present in the 'normal' aging brain? How do these changes differ from those seen in various types of dementia?

Links with radiology

In the two CT brain scans shown in Figures 12.2 and 12.3 of elderly people, what pathological changes can be seen and what structures may be affected? Which scan matches which of the following descriptions?

Patient A presented with a history of severe self-neglect and marked difficulty in planning. Patient B presented with low mood and speech difficulties.

■ Further reading and references ■

ATKINSON J H, GRANT I 1994 Natural history of neuropsychiatric manifestations of HIV disease. Psychiatric Clinics of North America 17(1): 17–33

BRAAK H, BRAAK E, BOHL J 1993 Staging of Alzheimer-related cortical destruction. European Neurology 33(6): 403–8

COLLINGE J, PALMER M S 1993 Prion diseases in humans and their relevance to other neurodegenerative diseases. Dementia 4(3–4): 178–85

EVANS M 1994 Dementia. In: Green B H (ed) Psychiatry in General Practice. Kluwer Academic Publishers, Lancaster

FLINT A J 1994 Epidemiology and comorbidity of anxiety disorders in the elderly. American Journal of Psychiatry 151(5): 640–9

GANZINI L, WALSH J R, MILLAR S B 1993 Drug-induced depression in the aged. What can be done? Drugs and Aging 3(2): 147–58

GREEN B H, COPELAND J R M, DEWEY M E et al. 1992 Risk factors for depression in old age. Acta Psychiatrica Scandinavica 86(3): 213–17

GREEN B H, DEWEY M E, COPELAND J R M et al. 1994 Risk factors for recovery and recurrence of depression in the elderly. International Journal of Geriatric Psychiatry 9: 789–795

LESSER I M, MILLER B L, SWARTZ J R, BOONE K B,

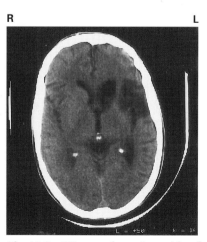

Fig. 12.2 CT scan of a patient with a fronto-parietal lobe infarction.

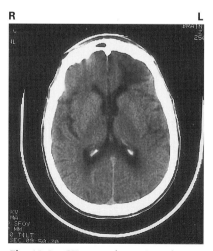

Fig. 12.3 CT scan of a patient showing a frontal lobe infarction.

MEHRINGER C M, MENA I 1993 Brain imaging in late-life schizophrenia and related psychoses. Schizophr-Bull. 19(4): 773–82

OLD AGE DEPRESSION INTEREST GROUP 1993 How long should the elderly take antidepressants? A double-blind placebo-controlled study of continuation/prophylaxis therapy with dothiepin. British Journal of Psychiatry 162: 175–82

NORDBERG A 1993 Clinical studies in Alzheimer patients with positron emission tomography. Behav-Brain-Res 30; 57(2): 215–24

PARKES C M 1964 The effects of bereavement on physical and mental health: a study of the case records of widows. British Medical Journal ii: 274–279

PRICE B H, GURVIT H, WEINTRAUB S, GEULA C, LEIMKUHLER E, MESULAM M 1993 Neuropsychological patterns and language deficits in 20 consecutive cases of autopsy-confirmed Alzheimer's disease. Archives of Neurology 50(9): 931–7

PROHOVNIK I, DWORK A J, KAUFMAN M A, WILLSON N 1993 Alzheimer-type neuropathology in elderly schizophrenia patients. Schizophr-Bull 19(4): 805–16

WHITEHOUSE P J 1993 Cholinergic therapy in dementia. Acta-Neurol-Scand-Suppl. 149: 42–5

Resources

Alzheimer's Disease Society,
2nd Floor,
Gordon House,
10 Greencoat Place,
London SW1P 1PH
Tel: 0171 306 0606

Age Concern,
Astral House,
1268 London Road,
Norbury,
London SW16 4ER
Tel: 0181 679 8000

Carers National Association,
20–25 Glasshouse Yard,
London EC1A HJS
Tel: 0171 490 8818

Compassionate Friends,
53 North Street,
Bristol BS3 1EN
Tel: 01272 539639

Counsel & Care (advice & help for older people),
Twyman House,
16 Bonny Street,
London NW1 9PG
Tel: 0171 485 1566

Crossroads,
10 Regent Place,
Rugby,
Warwickshire CV21 2PN
Tel: 01788 573653

CRUSE – Bereavement Care
Cruse House,
126 Sheen Road,
Richmond,
Surrey TW9 1UR
Tel: 0181 940 4818
Fax: 0181 940 7638
Cruse has 94 local branches and provides individual and group counselling. Cruse has a 'Bereavement Line' which provides a direct link to a counsellor: Mon-Fri from 9.30 a.m. to 5.00 p.m. Tel: 0181 332 7227

Help the Aged,
St. James Walk,
London EC1R 0BE
Tel: 0171 253 0253

National Association of Widows,
54–57 Alison Street,
Digbeth,
Birmingham B5 5TH
Tel: 0121 643 8348

Seniorline (Help the Aged)
Freephone 0800 289404.

Mental retardation

Mental retardation involves an impairment of intellect and learning ability of congenital origin. Causes may be genetic or environmental and have major implications for preventive medical practice and the ethical behaviour of health professionals. The relevance to psychiatry is the demonstration of how brain function can be affected by various congenital factors, how these may make psychiatric illness more likely, e.g. through epilepsy, and the impact on family function.

Contents

Causes

General intelligence, as measured by such things as IQ tests, is normally distributed in the population, and as a continuum may be assumed to have a polygenic inheritance (Fig. 13.1). However, environmental and genetic factors may act to reduce intelligence to abnormally low levels. Other factors may impair specific skills like reading only or language development.

Genetic causes

The classic chromosomal cause of mental retardation is Down syndrome, first described by Dr Langdon Down in 1866. The syndrome is usually caused by trisomy 21, but may rarely be due to a translocation (parts of damaged chromosomes are re-joined in an abnormal way). Table 13.1 shows the clinical features of Down syndrome (Fig. 13.2). Other autosomal causes include trisomy 13 (Patau syndrome), trisomy 18 (Edward syndrome) and deletion of part of chromosome 5 as in the 'cri-du-chat' syndrome. Sex chromosome abnormalities are also associated with retardation. Fragile-X syndrome, Klinefelter (XXY), Turner (XO), the XYY and the XXX syndrome are examples. Fragile-X syndrome is the second commonest known cause of mental retardation in males. Table 13.2 shows the clinical features of Fragile-X. Fragile-X carrying women may have some symptoms — reduced intellectual ability, poor muscle tone, prominent ears and long faces.

Single genes are causes of such conditions as tuberose sclerosis (autosomal dominant inheritance). In tuberose sclerosis tumours in the brain may cause epilepsy and cognitive impairment. Other autosomal dominant causes include Sturge-

Table 13.1   Clinical features of Down syndrome
• Oblique eye folds • Small, flattened skull • Large tongue • Broad hands with stumpy fingers • Single transverse palm crease • High cheek bones • Small height • Squint • Brushfield spots on the iris • Abnormal finger and toe prints • Cryptorchidism • Straight pubic hair • Congenital cardiac defects • Early dementia • Hypothyroidism

Table 13.2   Clinical features of Fragile-X syndrome
• Large, floppy ears • Protruding jaw • Macro-orchidism • Elongated face

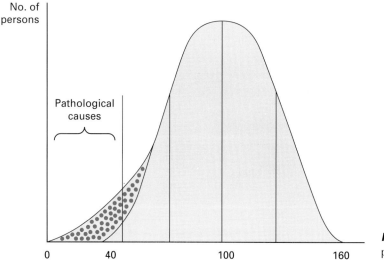

Fig. 13.1   The distribution of IQ in the population.

Weber syndrome (angiomatous malformation within the skull) and neurofibromatosis, where intracranial neuromas may occur. There are numerous autosomal recessive conditions such as phenylketonuria, galactosaemia, Hurler's disease and Niemann-Pick disease.

Other causes

The causes of some conditions are as yet unknown. Autism has been linked to Fragile-X syndrome, but this can account for only a small percentage of children with the condition. Early childhood autism is characterised by autistic aloneness, failure to make relationships, difficulties in perceiving certain sounds and images, overactivity or hyperkinesis in childhood ·and hypoactivity in adolescence, an 'obsessive desire for the maintenance of sameness', ritualistic behaviour, echolalia and pronoun reversal (e.g. using 'you' instead of 'I').

Intrauterine infection with syphilis, rubella, toxoplasmosis, influenza and cytomegalovirus can cause retardation. HIV infection acquired perinatally may present with a dementia-like illness in the early years of life. In this the fruits of early developmental milestones may be lost or never gained at all.

Other causes include kernicterus, obstetric instrumental brain damage, perinatal hypoxia and hydrocephalus.

Epidemiology

The specific causes of retardation are numerous and well-studied. Nevertheless, the majority of people with retardation cannot be given a specific cause for their condition. Why do you think this is?

Table 13.3 shows some how common various

Table 13.3 Epidemiology of mental retardation

Condition	Incidence
Down syndrome	1/660 live births in mothers aged 20 1/50 live births in mothers aged over 45
Fragile-X syndrome	1/1000 men
Klinefelter syndrome	1/1400 live births
XXX syndrome	1/1600 live births
Turner syndrome	1/3300 live births
Edward syndrome	1/3500 live births
Patau syndrome	1/7600 live births
Phenylketonuria	1/14 000 live births
Tuberose sclerosis	1/20 000 live births

causes of retardation are in the population. Among patients with IQs less than 50, about a third have Down syndrome, while 10–20% of retarded males have Fragile-X syndrome.

Psychiatry and mental retardation

The organic brain abnormalities which underlie mental retardation also predispose to epilepsy and to psychiatric illness. Whereas epilepsy affects less than 1% of all children, children with IQs of less than 50 are 40 times as likely to suffer from fits. About 10% of mentally retarded adults have had a fit in the previous year. Rates of psychiatric illness are also higher in the retarded compared to the general population. Perhaps as many as 30% of mentally retarded adults have a mental disorder. Alcoholism and drug abuse are very rare.

Failing to make the correct diagnosis of a mental illness and attributing abnormal speech and behaviour to mental retardation itself may lead to a per-

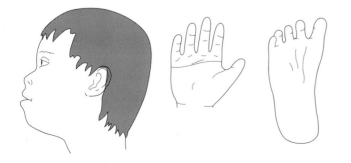

Fig. 13.2 The face, hand and foot in Down syndrome.

son not receiving the necessary and correct treatment for their illness. Drug treatment in this population is just as useful as in any other.

The presentation of the illness may, however, be modified by the degree of mental impairment. Affective disorders may present in terms of increased or reduced motor activity rather than specific complaints of sadness or elation. Altered eating and sleeping patterns, sexual indiscretions, mood lability, self-harm and attacks on others may all be signs. Schizophrenia may present with bizarre behaviour, poverty of thought, thought blocking, mannerisms and preoccupation with internal fantasy (although care is needed to distinguish this from normal fantasy).

Various organic processes can overlie the original mental retardation. Cognitive decline in a Down person must raise the suspicion of a superimposed dementia. Epilepsy (or anti-epileptics!) may cause confusional states. Self-harm may be a manifestation of out-of-control phenylketonuria.

Treatment options

Most mentally retarded people live at home. The family is their main support. Community resources, including highly trained teachers in regular schools, special schools, community adult training day centres, community nurses, specialist social workers and occupational therapists, may help support the family in their caring task. Because retarded people are significantly more vulnerable to psychiatric disorder than non-retarded people, access to psychiatric treatment is of high importance. Family doctors have a key role in coordinating medical care for this group of people.

Conventional antidepressants and antipsychotics may lead to significant improvements in mood and behaviour in psychiatrically ill retarded people.

Relatively selective serotononergic antidepressants (such as fluoxetine and clomipramine) have proved particularly useful in the treatment of compulsive and stereotyped behaviour in autistic patients.

Difficult behaviours, such as aggression, may respond to psychological interventions designed to discover triggers of such behaviour. Drug treatments with antipsychotics or antidepressants and mood stabilisers, such as carbamazepine and lithium, may be useful if coexisting psychiatric

disorder is present. Aggression, particularly episodic aggression, may be a feature of epileptic activity and may require antiepileptic medication. Paradoxically, hyperactivity disorders in retarded children may respond to stimulants such as methylphenidate.

CASE HISTORY 1

John was taken to his family doctor by his mother when he was aged 19. His mother had become concerned about him because for the past 2 months he had refused to leave the house and had started hoarding old newspapers and magazines. He kept these in strict date sequence on top of and behind cupboards, radiators and wardrobes. He had also taken to giggling inappropriately and making faces at thin air.

He had attended a comprehensive school and been part of a class of 35. He left school at the age of 16 but he had never learned to read or write properly and he could only do simple mental arithmetic. He enjoyed watching cartoons or motoring programmes on television. He had an amazing ability to recall details of vehicles and enjoyed talking about them at length, although other people found his conversation repetitive and dull. He had no friends and only a few acquaintances. He had never been able to find a job, although he dreamt of being a racing driver.

In what way is John different from most people?

John differs in two ways: he has a persistently low level of intelligence and recently has developed signs of mental illness. The details of his case are incomplete, but they do point towards various difficulties: coping with schoolwork, socialising with peers and restricted areas of interest. These would be consistent with mild mental retardation, although the history above gives no hint as to the aetiology of this. It is possible for mildly retarded people to make their way through regular school, although they perhaps do not progress to such levels as their peers and may find difficulties in gaining employment in a very competitive and technologically orientated job market. In school it is important to recognise learning difficulties so that teaching strategies can be adjusted to maximise the individual's potential. It is important to distinguish between specific learning difficulties, e.g. numerical skills, and more global cognitive disabilities.

Against the background of mild mental retardation, John is exhibiting some signs of mental disorder such as social withdrawal, compulsive hoarding and possible hallucinations which might make a doctor consider whether John was developing schizophrenia or had an affective disorder. Certainly a referral would be appropriate to either an adult psychiatrist or a psychiatrist specialising in learning disability.

CASE HISTORY 2

Anne was brought to her family doctor by her foster mother and her social worker, who had been increasingly concerned about her for some weeks. Anne was now aged 4. She had begun to walk and talk at the appropriate ages. Six months ago she had even begun to read simple texts. Now, however, she had stopped speaking in sentences and seemed to have difficulty comprehending speech. Her foster mother found it increasingly difficult to get Anne to concentrate on anything for more than a few minutes, whereas previously her concentration had been very good. The doctor watched Anne playing with the toys in her surgery and noticed that Anne was really quite clumsy. This too was something new.

What is the main problem described here?

Ann is a 4-year-old girl who was making good progress developmentally. In recent months this progress has not only been halted, but has actually reversed.

How does this differ from conventional mental retardation?

Conventionally in mental retardation certain skills and abilities are either never acquired or acquired with great difficulty. Anne's problem is almost the reverse of this — here skills once acquired are being lost, as in dementia.

Table 13.4 Causes of dementia in childhood

- HIV encephalopathy (commonest worldwide cause of childhood dementia)
- Wilson's disease (autosomal recessive inheritance, associated with abnormal movements, potentially reversible)
- Huntington's chorea (autosomal dominant inheritance, abnormalities of chromosome 4, predictive testing available)
- Leucodystrophies
- Subacute sclerosing panencephalitis (late complication of measles, more common in boys, typical EEG changes)
- Rett's syndrome
- Pervasive developmental disorders

What could be causing Anne's cognitive decline?

Normal development sometimes ebbs and flows. There may be a plateau in the development of new skills or the child may even revert or regress to more childish ways when stressed or physically unwell.

In Anne's case though the reversal is alarming — good receptive and expressive language skills seem to have disappeared, and the conjunction with motor signs such as clumsiness suggests a process affecting the CNS in some way (Table 13.4).

The doctor enquired about Anne's family history from the social worker and learnt that Anne's father was unknown. Her mother was, however, known to social services as an intravenous drug addict who had shared needles with others. On the basis of this information the doctor formed a hypothesis as to what was wrong with Anne. What hypothesis do you think this was and how would you investigate it if you were the doctor?

LEARNING POINTS

Mental retardation
- General intelligence, as measured by IQ tests, is roughly normally distributed in the population.
- One of the most common identified causes of retardation is Down syndrome — about a third of moderately retarded people have it. About 10–20% of retarded males have Fragile-X syndrome.
- About 30% of mentally retarded adults have a mental disorder.
- About 30% of mentally retarded adults have epilepsy.

Self-assessment

MCQs

1 Causes of mental retardation which affect more than 1/10 000 live male births include:
   a Down syndrome
   b Huntington's chorea
   c Fragile-X syndrome
   d enteroviruses
   e Wilson's disease

2 Compared to people with an IQ of 100 or more, people with learning disability:
   a have an equal chance of developing mental illness
   b are several times more likely to have epilepsy
   c when mentally ill require smaller doses of psychotropic medication
   d are more likely to be infertile
   e are significantly more likely to be violent

3 Active prevention of mental retardation in first pregnancies is currently possible for:
   a phenylketonuria
   b cytomegalovirus
   c toxoplasmosis
   d Hurler's syndrome
   e trisomy 18

4 In Down syndrome:
   a the 'severity' of facial stigmata predict poor intelligence and reduced self-sufficiency later in life
   b epileptic phenomena are exceedingly rare
   c the majority of births occur in mothers aged 30–39
   d receptive language ability declines with age

5 Learning disability:
   a is present in about 3% of the population
   b caused by trisomy 18 is known as 'cri-du-chat'
   c due to phenylketonuria is caused by a deficiency of phenylalanine
   d is associated with an increased tendency to epileptic fits
   e in a person means that psychotherapy cannot be offered as a treatment option

Short answer questions

1 List *five* causes of fetal malformations (other than alcohol or prescribed drugs).
2 List the clinical features of the foetal alcohol syndrome.

3 List *three* different mechanisms by which genetic abnormalities are transmitted and types of mental retardation associated with these.

MCQ answers

1 a = T, b = F, c = T, d = F, e = F
2 a = F, b = T, c = F, d = T, e = F
3 a = T, b = F, c = T, d = F, e = F
4 a = F, b = F, c = F, d = T
5 a = T, b = F, c = F, d = T, e = F

Short answers questions — answers

1 Ionising radiation, maternal disease (e.g. diabetes mellitus), maternal infection (e.g. rubella), pollution (e.g. dioxins), genetic and dietary deficiencies or excesses amongst others.
2 Intrauterine growth retardation, failure to thrive, short stature, mild to moderate mental retardation, microcephaly, thin upper lip, small eyes, maxillary hypoplasia, hyperactivity and others.
3 Dominant gene, e.g. tuberose sclerosis
   Deleted autosome, e.g. 'cri-du-chat'
   Trisomy, e.g. Edward syndrome
   Others include: recessive gene, extra autosome, extra sex chromosome, deleted sex chromosome and sex linked recessive gene.

Explorations

Sources listed in the 'Further reading and reference' section will help you with the following.

Links with obstetrics

What routine aspects of antenatal care are designed to prevent mental retardation? What aspects of perinatal and postnatal care are designed to prevent mental retardation?

Links with paediatrics and medicine

Besides the CNS, what other organ systems can be affected in Down syndrome? How can this be treated? What are the main causes of mortality in Down syndrome?

Links with psychology and sociology

How do parents react to their own mentally retarded offspring a) before, b) just after and c) years after the diagnosis is confirmed? How does the arrival of a mentally retarded child affect its siblings?

Further reading and references

COLLACOTT R A, COOPER S A, McGROTHER C 1992 Differential rates of psychiatric disorders in adults with Down syndrome compared with other mentally handicapped adults. British Journal of Psychology 161: 671–674

DUPONT A, VOETH M, VIDEBECH P 1986 Mortality and life expectancy of Down syndrome in Denmark. Journal of Mental Deficiency Research 30: 111–120

GATH A 1973 The school-age siblings of mongol children. British Journal of Psychiatry 123: 161–167

GATH A 1977 The impact of an abnormal child upon the parents. British Journal of Psychiatry 130: 405–410

HALL S M 1992 Congenital toxoplasmosis. British Medical Journal 305: 291–297

LANGDON DOWN J 1866 Observations on an ethnic classification of idiots. Clinical lectures and reports of the London Hospital 3: 259–262

KANNER L, EISENBERG L 1955 Notes on the follow-up studies of autistic children. In: Koch P H, Zubin J (eds) Psychopathology of Childhood. Grune & Stratton, New York

MULTIDISCIPLINARY WORKING GROUP 1992 Pre-natal screening for toxoplasmosis in the UK. Royal College of Obstetricians and Gynaecologists, London

MURDOCH J C 1985 Congenital heart disease as a significant factor in the morbidity of children with Down syndrome. Journal of Mental Deficiency Research 29: 147–151

PATAU K et al 1960 Multiple congenital anomaly caused by an extra autosome. Lancet 1: 790–793

REID A S 1982 The psychiatry of mental handicap. Blackwell Scientific Publications, London

THOMPSON C, WESTWELL P, VINEY D 1994 Psychiatric aspects of human immunodeficiency virus in childhood & adolescence. In: Rutter, Taylor and Hersov (eds.), Child and adolescent psychiatry. Blackwell Scientific Publications, Oxford, pp 711–719

TURK J 1992 The Fragile-X syndrome. On the way to a behavioural phenotype. British Journal of Psychiatry 160: 24–35

VERNON P E 1960 Intelligence and attainment tests. University of London Press, London

WING J K 1966 Early childhood autism. Pergamon Press, London

Resources

Down Syndrome Association,
155 Mitcham Road,
London SW17 9PG

National Autistic Society,
276 Willesden Lane,
London NW2 5RB
Tel: 0181 451 1114

14

Psychotherapy

Psychotherapy and counselling are 'talking cures' in which mental disorders can be treated over time and in which the relationship with the therapist is often of vital importance. Although psychotherapy is often a viable alternative to physical treatment, physical and psychological treatments can also be combined. In depression particularly patients may have a better prognosis if both kinds of treatment are used.

Contents

Psychological treatments

Psychotherapies include:

- behavioural therapy
- cognitive therapy
- cognitive-behavioural therapy
- group therapy
- family therapy
- interpersonal psychotherapy
- psychoanalysis
- counselling and many others.

There are so many different styles of psycho-therapy and counselling that it is impossible to describe them all. The differences in style, content and duration of therapies mean that it is very difficult to research the effectiveness of different therapies for specific conditions. This also makes it difficult to generalise from published research on any particular form of therapy.

Talking cures have been used for centuries, which attests to their popularity. Soranus of Ephesus, a physician working in the first century AD, talked to his patients and challenged the false ideas of people with depression. Nowadays, in cognitive therapy, therapists look for erroneous ways of thinking in depressed people and teach them to challenge these themselves. Holy men in all kinds of cultures have listened to the troubles of people who came to consult them and these people often derived comfort and reassurance from pouring out their heart.

There was much interest in the work of *Sigmund Freud* at the end of the nineteenth and beginning of the twentieth centuries. He believed that many mental disorders, particularly neuroses, arose from the unconscious, where they were attributed to ideas, memories or desires that could not be accepted by the conscious mind and were, therefore, repressed into the unconscious. Patients used to lie on Freud's couch in Vienna for an hour a day, every day, and recount whatever came into their minds (the method of so-called *free association*). Free association often led the patient to talking about traumas in their childhood that accounted, in part, for their current distress. Since the unconscious often works on a symbolic level, Freud also explored the unconscious by means of dream analysis. Patients would recount their dreams in detail

and together the patient and Freud would explore the symbolic meaning of the dream's content, often by asking the patient what ideas they associated with things in the dream.

CASE HISTORY 1

In her third session of therapy Anne brought along a dream that she had in the previous week. She had dreamt of entering a big house with a large hall and a wide staircase. Room by room Anne began exploring the place with the help of a guide. The ground floor and first floor boasted quite comfortable rooms with dark wood panelling and deep red curtains. The rooms were, nonetheless, cheery and bright and the sun streamed through the windows. However, in some dark corridors sections of flooring were sagging and her guide referred to rot in the fabric of the floor. On the first floor landing the guide pointed out a top floor to which he could not yet take her. She tried to see up the stairs and saw a brighter place where some golden girl was singing. Next the guide showed her some steps that led to the basement. A man and a woman lived there in the gloom. Anne felt that she did not want to go downstairs 'because of the things that happen there'.

What do you think that the therapist might make of this dream? Is it an optimistic dream or a pessimistic one? What could parts of the dream symbolise?

It is difficult to interpret dreams without knowing enough about the patient and the context of the dream. Dreams sometimes merely seem to repeat the previous day's events. In this case Anne could have been looking around an old house with an estate agent the day before and that might help explain elements of her dream. However, in this case the therapist discussed the dream's contents with Anne and together they decided that the dream was on the whole an optimistic one that was about Anne and her therapy. In the dream the house represented Anne's life, with the ground and first floor as her current life, which was largely a happy one although occasionally spoilt by periods of low mood (symbolised by the rot in dark corridors). The basement was her past, shrouded in darkness and unclear in detail. The top floor seemed to be a possible future. The language describing the top floor is optimistic: 'golden' and 'singing'.

The guide in the dream house was probably a representation of the therapist. If the therapist was to ask for more details about the guide this might give a chance to find out what Anne thought about him. In psychotherapy much attention is focused on these feelings which are often held to be the patient's *transference*. Transference involves the patient bringing their past experiences and emotions into therapy and transferring the qualities of significant past relationships onto the therapist. When these are recognised and interpreted properly it can help the patient gain control over feelings and ways of relating to others that may always have seemed overwhelming and mysterious before. Alexander and French (1946) called this 're-experiencing the old, unsettled conflict, but with a new ending' a corrective emotional experience.

CASE HISTORY 2

Mrs Davenport had been referred by her doctor to a psychologist. Mrs Davenport complained that she felt she was a 'worthless person' and that she felt 'guilty' that she could not be 'a better mother'.

The psychologist asked exactly why Mrs Davenport felt she was 'worthless'. She replied 'I was putting the washing out to dry this morning when the clothes line broke and all the washing fell onto the ground. It's the kind of thing that happens to me.' When asked why she needed to be a 'better mother' Mrs Davenport said, 'My 20-year-old son got his girlfriend pregnant, but he's not sorry about it. I should have taught him some values.'

How are the events that Mrs Davenport described linked to the way she feels?

It is difficult to see exactly how. Some events happen (the washing falls down, her son gets his girlfriend pregnant), Mrs Davenport thinks about these, draws some very large conclusions ('I'm worthless' and 'I should be a better mother') and feels low because of these ideas (or cognitions).

Cognitive therapy seeks to work on this link between cognitions and emotions. The work of Aaron T. Beck and colleagues focused on people with anxiety and depression. They concluded that in these disorders people have various negative automatic thoughts based on various cognitive errors. For instance, Mrs Davenport makes a giant leap of thought from her washing getting dirty to her being 'worthless'. This way of thinking may have roots in the past, but can be challenged and hopefully lead Mrs Davenport to draw different conclusions about herself. In the future, cognitive therapy would help her become skilled at finding alternatives to negative automatic thoughts. For example, in the case of the washing Mrs Davenport might think, 'The wind was strong and the washing line was old which was why it broke. I can buy a new washing line and I can wash the clothes again. I can cope with the unexpected.' Her therapist might ask her to keep a diary of her thoughts and feelings and ask her to record what alternative thoughts she found to her original negative thoughts. The diary could be reviewed during therapy sessions.

The structure of individual therapy

Psychotherapists generally give a structure to the therapy by ensuring that sessions are all of a similar length (usually about 50 minutes), are given regularly (say, once a week) and conducted in the same room at the same time of day by the same therapist. This agreement between therapist and client for a course of therapy is known as the *therapy contract*. Contact between the therapist and client between sessions or after therapy has ended is discouraged. These are the *boundaries* of therapy. A course of psychotherapy may be brief, e.g. 8 weeks, or long-term, e.g. 3 years.

Behaviour therapy

Behaviour therapy is usually employed when specific goals can be established, e.g. in a phobia of flying where the patient really wants to fly on holiday but cannot face the journey. In such phobias therapists often use *systematic desensitisation* using a *hierarchy* of stimuli. For instance, a person with a phobia of spiders may be presented with a dead spider in a jar at the end of the room (an *aversive stimulus*). At this stage the patient is taught how to relax in the presence of the spider. Having achieved this, the next aversive stimulus in the hierarchy is presented, e.g. a live spider in a jar at the end of the room. Relaxation is repeated and so on until the final stimulus in the hierarchy is presented, e.g. handling a spider, or in the case of the flying phobic taking a plane journey.

More complicated behaviour therapy programmes can be used to reward certain desired behaviours, e.g. hygiene or self-presentation skills in chronic schizophrenia, or appropriate seeking of help in deliberate self-harm patients, and deliberately not rewarding undesirable behaviours, e.g. violence or self-harm.

In obsessive-compulsive disorder, systematic desensitisation may be used. For instance, in compulsive handwashing the patient may be encouraged to handle increasingly dirty things and postpone washing by attempting to relax. The prevention of compulsions is often called *response prevention*. Clinical psychologists are often expert in the construction of behavioural therapy programmes.

Family therapy

This may be conducted by a family therapist who may work with the family together in a room separated from another by a one-way screen. Behind the screen a colleague or supervisor can watch the family and its interactions with each other and the therapist and feed back to the therapist in the next room via a telephone or audio ear piece.

Although psychiatric illness mainly affects an individual within a family, the family is usually affected by the consequences of the illness or may affect the prognosis of the illness by their actions. Hostile, over-involved and critical families may adversely affect relapse rates of schizophrenic members. Bulimia nervosa has been associated with families where there is excessive conflict and anorexia nervosa has been linked to rather repressed, controlled families, sometimes with 'distant' or uninvolved fathers. Various mental disorders have also been linked to abusive relationships within families, although evidence for this is often contested.

Family therapy seeks to establish and reflect back the family's structure and style of interacting and to change this style if it appears to be a problem. Because the family is a system of individuals rather than a single individual with a disorder, it has proved difficult to research the effectiveness of family therapy, but it has proved successful in a variety of mental disorders.

Group therapy

In group therapy a group of about six to eight people meet regularly with one to two therapists. Group therapy may involve a variety of therapeutic styles. Some groups may be supportive or educational, others may be interpretive and analytical. Groups may be formed of people with differing disorders, e.g. a day hospital group, or of people with similar problems, e.g. an eating disorders group. Patients in such groups often derive a feeling of mutual support and hope. New coping styles may be learned. From their own self-knowledge patients are particularly able to challenge other group members' defences. For instance, if a member of an alcohol abuse group projects all the blame for his heavy drinking onto his absent wife, a group peer may be more able than a therapist to confront him with the fact that it is he who is drinking too much, not his wife.

LEARNING POINTS

Psychological treatments

- Defence mechanisms are psychological devices used to prevent or reduce psychological discomfort. They include denial, projection, displacement and repression.
- Transference is a mechanism whereby people transfer emotions from one past setting to another. For instance, we may feel comfortable with a stranger because he or she reminds us or someone we previously knew and liked.
- Dreams can be useful tools in psychotherapy. They contain messages from the unconscious mind, often in a symbolic form. They need to be interpreted with care according to the context and experience of the patient.
- Cognitive therapy focuses on the thoughts associated with various emotions. For instance,

depression may be associated with various negative automatic thoughts such as 'I can't cope' or 'I'm useless'. Cognitive therapy seeks to challenge such thoughts and restructure them.

- Family therapy is used in a variety of mental disorders and focuses on the impact that they have on the family and the way that families can affect the illness. Family therapy seeks to identify dysfunctional interactions between family members and suggest alternative ways of behaving that may be tried within therapy sessions.
- Group therapy occurs in a group of about eight patients together with one or two therapists. Members of the groups support, encourage and challenge each other whilst the experienced therapist shapes the group's progress. Group therapy is useful in restructuring personal relationship behaviour and attitudes and can be used in a variety of disorders, e.g. alcoholism and eating disorders.

Self-assessment

MCQs

1 Appropriate psychotherapies for people with mental retardation include:
   a group therapy
   b family therapy
   c psychoanalysis
   d behavioural therapy
   e cognitive therapy

2 Classical ingredients of cognitive therapy include:
   a focusing on the transference
   b dream analysis
   c exposing psychological defence mechanisms
   d challenging erroneous ways of thinking
   e use of a diary

3 Behaviour therapy:
   a is not of use in obsessive-compulsive disorder
   b is used almost exclusively by approved social workers
   c may involve systematic desensitisation
   d may involve relaxation training
   e focuses on thoughts

Short answer questions

In the following vignettes think what you would say next to the patients during a long interview:

1 (A 47-year-old man with alcohol dependency) 'I went on a binge last weekend. I couldn't stop myself. I went in to celebrate a win on the horses, and I just had one after the other and before I knew it I was down again. Thinking about what I was going to do in the future. Thinking about how it's all my wife's fault. If she hadn't insisted that we move here I wouldn't have started work at Taylor's and I wouldn't have been made redundant. And then I wouldn't have an alcohol problem . . . .'

2 (A 20-year-old woman who presents with anxiety attacks) 'I've never told anybody this . . . (pause) . . . I am so ashamed about it . . . I . . . promise me that you'll never tell anybody . . . please?'

3 (A 40-year-old woman recalling her father who died during her childhood.) So I never really knew him when I grew up . . . he was just this smiling face when I was little . . . and ice creams and trips out. I remember him rowing me down the river on a boat . . . (tears begin to form in her eyes) . . . and . . . (she pauses and cannot continue speaking).

MCQ answers

1 a = T, b = T, c = F, d = T, e = T
2 a = F, b = F, c = F, d = T, e = T
3 a = F, b = F, c = T, d = T, e = F

Explorations

Sources listed in the 'Further reading and reference' section will help you with the following.

Links with public health

Local health purchasers are keen to set up a variety of therapies for primary care including a psychotherapy and counselling service. They only have a limited budget for mental health. Investing in psychotherapy and counselling will mean that some resources will have to be diverted from elsewhere. Imagine you are an adviser to the purchasers. What evidence is there that psychotherapy is an effective treatment for a mental disorder like depression? Is any therapy particularly useful? Which therapy style might be the most cost-effective?

Links with medicine

How many cases referred to general medical clinics have a strong psychological component? What is somatisation? How can psychotherapy or counselling skills help doctors manage these patients sympathetically and effectively? What percentage of people on general medical wards have depressive symptoms? How might these symptoms be detected and treated? What contribution to recovery might psychotherapy or counselling make?

Further reading and references

ALEXANDER F, FRENCH T M 1946 Psychoanalytic therapy. Ronald Press Co., New York

BALINT M 1964 The Doctor, his Patient and the Illness. Pitman Medical, Kent

BECK A T, RUSH A J, SHAW B F, EMERY G 1979 Cognitive therapy of depression. Guilford Press, New York

BERGIN A E, GARFIELD S L 1994 Handbook of psychotherapy and behaviour change, 4th edn. Wiley, Chichester.

BOWLBY J 1984 Attachment, 2nd edn. Pelican, London

GREEN B H 1995 Creating Rapport. In: Green (ed) Psychiatry in General Practice. Kluwer Academic Publishers, London

HALEY J 1986 Uncommon therapy. W W Norton & Co, New York

HAWTHORNE K, SALKOVSKIS P M, KIRK J, CLARK D M 1989 Cognitive behaviour therapy for psychiatric problems. A practical guide. Oxford Medical Publications. Oxford

HOBSON R F 1985 Forms of feeling. The heart of psychotherapy. Tavistock, London

MALAN D H 1979 Individual psychotherapy and the science of psychodynamics. Butterworths, London

PECK M S 1978 The road less travelled. Simon & Schuster, New York

STAFFORD-CLARK D 1965 What Freud really said. Macdonald, London

STORR A 1979 The Art of Psychotherapy. Martin, Secker & Warburg, London

Psychotherapy in literature

Davies R The Deptford Trilogy

15

Physical treatments

Physical treatments used in psychiatry today include drugs, electroconvulsive therapy (ECT), and psychosurgery.

Contents

Advances in physical treatments

In the 1950s new antipsychotic drugs began to be used in preference to surgery because they were more efficacious in schizophrenia, had fewer side-effects and, unlike iatrogenic brain damage, were reversible.

Before these drugs a variety of treatments were attempted that nowadays seem bizarre. Padded cells, straitjackets, insulin induced comas, purging, cold wet blanket baths, spinning chairs, colonic irrigation and magnetic fields have all been employed in the desperate search for a cure. No doubt some patients responded to a placebo effect and others became well spontaneously, as with physical illnesses. These good responses were used anecdotally to boost the claims of such odd treatments.

The advent of the French drug *chlorpromazine* in 1952 showed that there could be a drug with a specific antipsychotic effect. Patients with schizophrenia who had been hospitalised for many years were transformed within weeks of the new treatment.

Electroconvulsive therapy (ECT), first used in 1938, and the development of *tricyclic antidepressants* revolutionised the prognosis of depression.

These new physical treatments enabled community care and the decanting of thousands of patients from the old county asylums. Before the new physical treatments, florid psychotic states in schizophrenia were often life-long and depressed patients sometimes endured the unremitting burden of their illness for years.

Psychosurgery

Surgery to areas such as the frontal or temporal lobe is termed psychosurgery. Psychosurgery is rarely used nowadays but was once in vogue following pioneering work on frontal lobe surgery by Egaz Moniz, who won the Nobel Prize in 1948. Psychosurgery is often effective but is irreversible, so unwanted effects on moods or personality are permanent.

Psychosurgery is still performed on patients whose illnesses are severe and unresponsive to drugs, for example in patients with persistent, severe, life-dominating anxiety. Psychosurgery operations are rare now and in the UK number only in the order of tens per year and are performed in specialist centres.

Perhaps because of the over-use of psychosurgery in the past and mankind's intrinsic horror of mental illness, physical treatments for mental illness have acquired a frightening public image.

Future developments

Collecting scientific data about the efficacy of physical treatments against placebos has enabled a process of continual refinement and innovation.

Continuing research aims to replace established treatments with more ideal treatments that are safer, easier to comply with, more efficacious, non-addictive, more cost-effective and quicker-acting. New drugs are tested against the old standard treatments to establish these criteria. New antidepressants are rigorously tested against the old 'gold standard' antidepressants amitryptiline and imipramine. Newer antidepressants such as fluoxetine are safer in overdose and offer a more acceptable treatment to the patient. In recent years a new atypical antipsychotic, clozapine, has offered hope to patients with treatment-resistant schizophrenia. Based on this advance new safer, more effective antipsychotics are in development.

Antipsychotic drugs

Antipsychotic drugs are sometimes called neuroleptics or major tranquillisers. They are used in treating schizophrenia and in short-term control of psychotic states and abnormal behaviour. They are usually sedative.

Main pharmacological actions

The main group of antipsychotic drugs exert their effect by blocking dopamine receptors in the brain. Blockade of dopamine receptors also leads to side effects and, because cholinergic, histamine and noradrenergic receptors can also be affected, the side effects can be varied.

Routes of administration

Antipsychotic drugs can usually be given orally or

intramuscularly (for emergency control of disturbed behaviour) and also by long-term depot injections (which allow the drug to leach into the blood stream over a period of weeks). Antipsychotics are not usually given intravenously.

Common side-effects

Side-effects often depend on the type of neurotransmitter system affected. Over-sedation may arise from activity at histamine receptors. Dry mouth, blurred vision, nasal stuffiness, constipation and tremor occur because of anticholinergic effects at muscarinic receptors. Postural hypotension (particularly dangerous in the elderly) is due to peripheral and central alpha-adrenoceptor blockade. A reflex tachycardia and peripheral vasodilatation may lead to a concomitant hypothermia. Because of dopamine blockade in the hypothalamo-pituitary axis, prolactin levels rise dramatically (and may lead to lactation in females).

Other side-effects

- Jaundice due to intrahepatic stasis.
- Pigmentary changes in the skin and eyes (oculodermal melanosis).
- Photosensitivity.
- Movement disorders including acute dystonic reactions, restlessness (akathisia) and tardive dyskinesia.
- Bone marrow suppression.
- Lowering of the epileptic threshold.

Acute parkinsonian side-effects can be reversed by agents such as procyclidine (given 10 mg i.v. in acute dystonia, but otherwise given orally).

Interactions with other drugs

- Alcohol.
- CNS depressants, e.g. benzodiazepines, barbiturates.
- Antihypertensives.
- Levodopa.
- Antiepileptics.

Chlorpromazine: the first antipsychotic

Chlorpromazine was the first antipsychotic in widespread use in 1952. Its structure is similar to that of a phenothiazine. Its main clinical effect arises from its blockade of dopamine (D2) receptor sites. Chlorpromazine is a sedative and is particularly effective at controlling disturbed behaviour when given intramuscularly. Up to 80% of an oral dose of chlorpromazine is removed by the first-pass metabolism before it ever reaches the brain. There is no depot preparation. Intravenous administration may provoke a fatal arrythmia.

A typical dose regime for a young man with schizophrenia might be 150 mg of chlorpromazine 4 times a day. In an acute emergency where sedation is required a dose of 100–150 mg i.m. could be used. In older or smaller patients the dose must be altered.

Other typical antipsychotics

Haloperidol (a butyrophenone) was another early antipsychotic. It is less sedating, more potent and more likely to induce dystonic reactions than chlorpromazine. There is a depot preparation. Other butyrophenones include benperidol, droperidol and trifluperidol. Haloperidol is roughly 10 times more potent than chlorpromazine so that 10 mg of haloperidol produces the same effect of 100 mg of chlorpromazine.

Other phenothiazines include thioridazine, which is often used in the elderly, and trifluoperazine, which is often used in paranoid states.

Newer antipsychotics include sulpiride (a substituted benzamide which seems to have less potential for inducing movement disorders) and loxapine (a dibenzodiazepine).

Two drugs are mainly used as depot injections given into the gluteal region: fluphenazine given 12.5–100 mg every 2 to 5 weeks and thioxanthene given 50–300 mg every 2 to 4 weeks.

Treatment strategy

In terms of a strategy for using antipsychotics, the initial phase may, for example, begin with oral chlorpromazine or sulpiride. Over the next few days or weeks the clinician will titrate the dose up or down and might expect hallucinatory symptoms to cease and delusions to recede as insight returns. Maintenance of remission can be achieved using depot injections such as fluphenazine or thioxanthene. A once-monthly injection is better in compliance terms than an oral drug meant to be taken three times daily. Alterations to this strategy occur when there are side-effects that require the use of anti-Parkinsonian drugs, such as procyclidine, given concurrently or if there is treatment resistance (when ultimately clozapine might prove useful). Some units begin new patients on an initial short-acting injection of thioxanthene (rather than starting on an oral preparation) and then move to long-acting depot injections of the same drug.

Treatment resistance

About 20% of patients with schizophrenia are deemed to be treatment resistant after various first-line treatments have failed. Up to two-thirds of these resistant cases may respond to clozapine. Clozapine is an atypical antipsychotic given orally in a tightly-controlled treatment programme. One to two per cent of clozapine patients are prone to bone marrow failure and therefore the white-cell count is monitored weekly or fortnightly. If the white cell count falls significantly, the treatment is stopped whilst there is still sufficient marrow function to guarantee recovery. New drugs based on clozapine, but without potentially lethal side-effects, are on the horizon, thus offering the hope that all patients with schizophrenia will one day be effectively treated.

Antidepressant drugs

Tricyclics

Tricyclic antidepressants are so-called because of a three ring structure (Fig. 15.1). They can be expected to be successful in treating 70% of depressive episodes compared to a 30–50% placebo response. Examples of tricyclics include amitriptyline (introduced 1961), imipramine (1959) and dothiepin (1969). Dothiepin is the most frequently prescribed tricyclic in the UK.

The tricyclics' main effect occurs through inhibiting the re-uptake of monoamines from the synaptic cleft by the pre-synaptic neurone (Fig. 15.2). Monoamines involved include noradrenaline, serotonin and dopamine. The proven efficacy of tri-

cyclics led to the monoamine theory of depression: depression is secondary to a relative deficiency of monoamines in the synapse. Tricyclic antidepressants act by prolonging monoamine activity at the synapse.

Insomnia is resolved quickly (especially when the main dose of tricyclic is taken at bedtime) because of the tricyclics' sedative properties. However, improvement in mood lags behind improvement in sleep by some weeks. Gradually raising the daily drug dose to a certain threshold also seems to be important before tricyclics work.

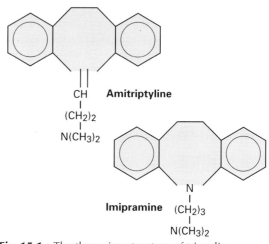

Fig. 15.1 The three ring structure of tricyclic antidepressants.

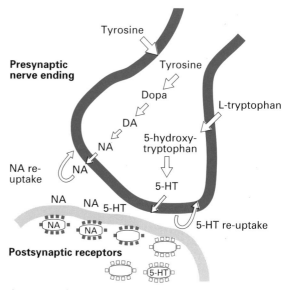

Fig. 15.2 The synapse.

Common reasons for the failure of tricyclic antidepressant therapy

- Inadequate dose.
- Not taken regularly by patient.
- Wrong diagnosis.
- Wrong drug type.

Side-effects of tricyclics

Most side-effects are caused by indiscriminate actions on various neurotransmitter systems. These side-effects make tricyclics less acceptable to some patients and considerably reduce patient compliance.

Anticholinergic side-effects

- Dry mouth.
- Blurred vision.
- Urinary retention.
- Constipation.
- Sweating.
- Confusion.

Adrenergic side-effects

- Postural hypotension.
- Tachycardia.
- Cardiac arrhythmias (may cause death in susceptible individuals and in overdose. Tricyclics used to cause 400 overdose deaths annually in the UK.)

Antihistaminic side-effects

- Drowsiness and sedation (particularly important to those who operate dangerous machinery or drive).

  Other side-effects include weight-gain (by stimulating appetite), hypomania, restlessness, rashes, photosensitivity, bone marrow suppression, nausea and impotence.

Contraindications to tricyclics

- Simultaneous prescription of irreversible mono-amine-oxidase inhibitors
- Heart block and recent myocardial infarction
- Prostatic hypertrophy (risk of precipitating acute urinary retention)
- Late pregnancy
- Narrow-angle glaucoma.

Newer tricyclics include maprotiline (1974) and lofepramine (1983). Lofepramine is less cardiotoxic than others.

CASE HISTORY 1

A 48-year-old woman with a 4-week history of low mood and biological features of depression was prescribed dothiepin 75 mg nocte by her doctor. Her doctor noted that an improvement in the patient's sleep began after 2 days. Two weeks later the doctor increased the dose of dothiepin to 100 mg nocte and 2 weeks after this the patient's mood had lifted significantly. She was maintained on dothiepin for the next 6 months and then gradually the drug was withdrawn by reducing the dose by 25 mg at intervals in out-patients.

Research indicates that 70% of patients who stop their antidepressants within 6 months of starting them relapse. Current opinion suggests that anti-depressant therapy should be maintained for up to a year at least and only then gradually withdrawn (monitoring for signs of relapse).

CASE HISTORY 2

A 54-year-old man with a 4-week history of low mood, insomnia and weight loss attended the psychiatry out-patient clinic. Despite his general practitioner's prescription of tricyclics 2 weeks ago the patient remained depressed. On mental state examination he revealed that he had been having suicidal ideas. He had been thinking of hanging himself. The ideas were suggested to him by derogatory second person auditory hallucinations.

Organic causes of his depressed mood and hallucinations had been fully excluded by his general practitioner.

Reasons why the tricyclic antidepressants appear not to have worked

The tricyclics may not have worked because they

have only had 2 weeks to work, they were prescribed at too low a dose, because the patient is only taking them intermittently or not at all or because the patient is not responding to this particular drug.

What is the likely diagnosis now?

The patient is suffering from a severe depression with psychotic features. Given his suicidal ideation and the severity of his illness he would require admission to monitor his well-being and compliance.

What physical treatments might be most suitable now?

He would probably benefit from electroconvulsive therapy (particularly effective for severe depression with psychotioc features, see below) and may also be given antipsychotic drugs.

Once this patient is euthymic, what physical treatments might be used to maintain his mental health?

In the long-term he would need continued antidepressant medication and/or lithium prophylaxis (see below) to avoid a recurrence of his depression.

Monoamine oxidase inhibitors (MAOIs)

MAOIs were introduced at about the same time as tricyclics. They were marginally less effective than tricyclics but were still better than placebo. They may have a special role in agoraphobia and panic disorder. The original MAOIs were irreversible inhibitors of MAO such as phenelzine and tranylcypromine. The latest MAOIs are reversible and called RIMAs (Reversible Inhibitors of Monoamine A) and have fewer side-effects and are just as effective as tricyclics. The original irreversible MAOIs inhibited both MAO-A and MAO-B and enhanced the amount of monoamine transmitters held in presynaptic storage vesicles. A variety of foods should be avoided by people taking irreversible MAOIs — mainly those which are high in tyramine — failure

to comply may lead to flushing, headache, hyperthermia and hypertensive encephalopathy, sometimes called the 'cheese reaction'.

Some food and drink to avoid with irreversible MAOIs

- Mature cheese.
- Yeast extracts.
- Textured vegetable protein.
- Dark beers.
- Chianti wine.
- Game that is high.
- Ripe avocado.
- Pickled herrings.

In addition there are drugs to avoid whilst taking MAOIs, particularly those drugs with sympathomimetic actions.

Some drugs to avoid with irreversible MAOIs

- Tricyclic antidepressants.
- SSRIs.
- L-dopa.
- Amphetamines.
- Cough and cold remedies (containing ephedrine and pseudoephedrine).
- Narcotic analgesics such as pethidine.
- Alcohol.

Because of these stringencies, MAOIs are seen as second-line treatments for depressive illness. It is important to remember that it takes at least 2 weeks for MAOIs to wash out of the patient after stopping them, so that patients should be warned to follow the above restrictions throughout the wash-out period.

Moclobemide is the first of a new generation of reversible inhibitors of monoamine oxidase A (RIMA) drugs. Because of the reversible nature of their enzyme, inhibition stringent diets and prescription modifications are not as important. The dietary restrictions above made old irreversible MAOIs unpopular with patients and doctors alike. RIMAs can be used in the elderly and are less problematic in overdose than tricyclics. The dose regimen for moclobemide is 300–600 mg per day.

Selective serotonin re-uptake inhibitors (SSRIs)

In the late 1980s SSRIs such as fluvoxamine and fluoxetine were first introduced. Because they are relatively specific in reducing re-uptake of serotonin, SSRIs lack many of the side-effects produced by tricyclic antidepressants. There are fewer anticholinergic and adrenergic side-effects. Cardiotoxicity is reduced and, as a result, SSRIs are much safer in overdose. Unwanted effects are largely attributable to serotonergic effects including nausea, diarrhoea, anxiety and appetite suppression. Examples of SSRIs include fluoxetine, paroxetine, sertraline and fluvoxamine. They all have differing chemical structures unlike the tricyclics (Fig. 15.3).

Fluoxetine and paroxetine are given once daily. The dose titration seen with tricyclics is generally not needed for fluoxetine (20 mg daily) or paroxetine (20 mg daily). SSRIs are not so sedative, but generally restorative effects on sleep precede antidepressive effects as with tricyclics. SSRIs usually work within 2–3 weeks. Experience suggests that patients need to be maintained on SSRIs even after their mood has responded. Unless this is mentioned by the doctor, patients tend to stop the treatment because they are feeling well again and, consequently, they may relapse. There is a current debate about just how long this maintenance therapy should be.

Where renal or hepatic function is impaired, SSRI prescribing may need to be altered. SSRIs may also reduce epileptic thresholds (as with other psychotropic drugs) and, therefore, provoke fits in susceptible individuals.

Recent work suggests that fluoxetine may also be useful in treating bulimia nervosa and premenstrual syndrome.

SSRIs and MAOIs are a potentially fatal combination causing hyperpyrexia. A wash-out period is recommended if switching from an SSRI to an MAOI (5 weeks for fluoxetine and 1 week for sertraline). If the switch is from an MAOI to an SSRI the wash-out period should be 2 weeks.

Mood stabilisers: lithium

Mood stabilising agents are used in bipolar affective disorder. Lithium carbonate (sometimes also available as lithium acetate) has been used as a first-line prophylactic agent in bipolar affective disorder for over 30 years. Other mood stabilisers include the anti-epileptic drugs carbamazepine and sodium valproate. These latter two drugs may be useful alternatives when lithium is contraindicated.

Lithium

Lithium carbonate is used mainly in the treatment of bipolar affective disorder. It is useful acutely in reducing hypomania and in maintaining remission. It is sometimes also used to prevent recurrences of depression in unipolar affective disorder.

In bipolar affective disorder, lithium reduces the frequency and severity of relapses of bipolar illness and reduces the suicide rate in treated individuals.

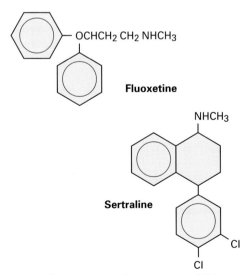

Fluoxetine

Sertraline

Fig. 15.3 Selective serotonin re-uptake inhibitors (SSRIs).

| CASE HISTORY 3 |

A 45-year-old man with a past psychiatric history of two manic episodes and one depressive episode in 2 years is currently maintained on 400 mg lithium carbonate b.d. with a serum level of 0.8. Serum levels of lithium need to be monitored regularly because of the ion's pharmacokinetics.

Pharmacokinetics

The serum half-life of lithium carbonate is 18–20 hours in young adults and 36–42 hours in the elderly. It has a low therapeutic index which means that serum concentration must be regularly monitored to keep within a therapeutic range of 0.6–0.8 mmol/l. Above 1.2 mmol/l toxic effects happen. Concentrations above 2.00 mmol/l may be fatal. 12% of patients who overdose on lithium die.

The serum level of lithium is linearly related to the ingested dose.

Lithium in its ionic form is naturally hydrophilic and is distributed mainly in intra- and extra-cellular fluid (not body fat). It is excreted by the kidney and thus good renal function is an essential to its prescription. If renal function is compromised then toxic levels of lithium can result.

Signs of lithium toxicity

- Anorexia.
- Nausea and diarrhoea.
- Tinnitus.
- Ataxia.
- Dysarthria.
- Drowsiness.
- Convulsions.
- Coma and death.

Management of high serum levels

The initial management of high serum levels may involve simply stopping lithium therapy for a few days and readjusting the dosage, but with higher levels osmotic or alkaline diuresis or peritoneal dialysis or haemodialysis may be necessary.

Baseline investigations

Before starting lithium therapy various baseline investigations need to be done:

- full blood count
- urea and electrolytes
- serum creatinine (provides an indication of glomerular filtration rate)
- thyroid function tests
- ECG.

Side-effects of lithium therapy

Early
- Nausea.
- Diarrhoea.
- Thirst.
- Polyuria.
- Fine tremor.
- Metallic taste.

Late
- Weight gain.
- Leucocytosis.
- Renal damage.
- ECG changes (T-wave inversion and QRS complex widening which may reverse once lithium is stopped).
- Hypothyroidism. In up to 15% of women taking lithium, hypothyroidism becomes a complication. It is, therefore, essential to have some baseline measurement of thyroid function. If hypothyroidism does occur it is often better to add in thyroid hormone replacement therapy rather than stop lithium.

Lithium use in young women

Lithium may have teratogenic effects if administered during pregnancy, specifically Ebstein's anomaly (cardiac malformation) and neural tube malformations if given during early pregnancy. Cyanosis, bradycardias and foetal death may occur if lithium is given in the last few weeks of pregnancy. Nursing mothers on lithium secrete lithium in breast milk. Patients at risk of becoming pregnant must be warned of these risks.

Interactions of lithium

Lithium interacts unfavourably with thiazide diuretics, aminoglycoside antibiotics and NSAIDs (because NSAIDs potentiate antidiuretic hormone).

Anxiolytics and hypnotics

Anxiolytics are those drugs such as benzodiazepines given to allay anxiety. Hypnotics are given to induce sleep and include such compounds as benzodiazepines, chloral hydrate, barbiturates and zopiclone. Chloral hydrate has been used since the 1890s and is still in use, but barbiturates, because of their addictiveness, are rarely used nowadays.

Anxiolytics and hypnotics are less in vogue today than 10 or 20 years ago. In 1981 it was estimated that 10% of men and 20% of women would take benzodiazepines at least once during the year. Problems with tolerance, dependence and withdrawal have forced many doctors to reconsider their prescribing habits. If the doctor suspects that there is an underlying depressive illness, insomnia may be better treated by antidepressants rather than hypnotics. Other insomnias may respond more to a 'sleep hygiene programme' which seeks to promote rest-inducing factors and reduce sleep-damaging factors.

Factors promoting sleep

- Exercise during day.
- Warm bath at bedtime.
- Milky drinks.
- Bedtime snack.
- 'Soft' music before bed.
- Relaxation tapes/exercises.

Factors adversely affecting sleep

- Caffeine in tea, coffee and soft drinks.
- Alcohol (although may induce sleep alcohol withdrawal promotes waking).
- Street drugs, e.g. amphetamines.
- Heavy meals.
- Withdrawal from short-acting benzodiazepines.

Benzodiazepines

Benzodiazepines act by making nerve cells more receptive to gamma-amino-butyric acid (GABA), an inhibitory neurotransmitter. Benzodiazepines therefore damp down neural activity and reduce cerebral excitation. They are useful in pre-anaesthetic sedation and in aborting epileptic fits.

Benzodiazepines are well absorbed when given orally, rectally or intravenously. Virtually all are metabolised by the liver by oxidation and conjugation. Benzodiazepine metabolites are often phar-

macologically active too (and may have longer half-lives).

Diazepam has a half-life of 20–30 hours, but its active metabolite, desmethyldiazepam, has a half-life of nearly 36–200 hours.

Benzodiazepines produce tolerance and dependence. The shorter the half-life is the more addictive the benzodiazepine. Once courses of benzodiazepines are stopped there is often rebound anxiety and rebound insomnia (as the brain tries to adjust to the sudden absence of a cerebral depressant). Withdrawal effects also include epileptic fits. Benzodiazepines suppress rapid eye movement sleep (REM sleep) and patients in withdrawal may complain of very vivid dreams because of a rebound REM phenomenon. Other withdrawal symptoms include: depersonalisation, perceptual distortions, panic attacks, craving, headache, muscle stiffness, formication, hypersensitivity, ataxia, muscle twitches, dysphagia, diarrhoea, nausea, vomiting, palpitations, hyperventilation, flushing, sweating, skin rash/itching and influenza-like symptoms amongst others. In order to reduce these effects patients are often weaned off short-acting agents onto long-acting ones which are gradually tailed down to zero.

Benzodiazepines may inhibit the mourning process if given in the acute phases of grief and also have cognitive side-effects impairing the formation of new memories.

Care is, therefore, taken to avoid medium- or long-term prescribing of these drugs. Their routine use in hospital is to be deplored since many patients have become addicted after short introductory spells on them in hospital.

However, discounting the many negative attributes of benzodiazepines, they are potent anxiolytics and no compound or psychological therapy comes close in rapid alleviation of anxiety. They are rarely fatal in overdose.

Electroconvulsive therapy (ECT)

Iatrogenically induced seizures have been used to treat depression since the early years of the twentieth century. Fits induced by smelling camphor or through injections of metrazol had been noted to abort depressive episodes. However, such methods of inducing fits were not without risk and it was not until Cerletti and Bini introduced ECT in Rome in 1938 that the way opened for a safer method. ECT nowadays is used to induce modified fits (modified in that muscle relaxants and short-acting anaesthetics are used). To induce the fit electrodes are placed bilaterally and a small pulsed current passed through the skull and brain. A modified generalised fit follows.

Without muscle relaxation, simultaneously contracting opposing muscle groups during the tonic phase can cause fractures of long bones and vertebrae. Anaesthetics used to induce unconsciousness make the procedure more tolerable.

ECT is rapidly effective in severe depression and is often the treatment of choice for depression with psychotic features. For such cases it is superior to antidepressants. The rapidity is valuable since acutely depressed individuals may stop eating and drinking (secondary to nihilistic delusions for example) and their lives may be at risk. ECT also rapidly reduces very real suffering. ECT treatments may be given twice a week for 6–8 weeks. Resolution of depression is rapid, but further improvement often continues through the course.

The induced fit is crucial to the therapeutic properties of ECT. Drugs which increase fit threshold (such as diazepam) impair its efficacy. Modified fits should be bilateral and last for about 30 seconds. Electrodes placed bilaterally seem more effective than electrodes placed unilaterally.

In terms of efficacy ECT has been repeatedly shown to resolve depressive illness more quickly and in more people than tricyclics or MAOIs (Fig. 15.4). It is particularly useful in severe depression where there are psychotic features. Given that there is a high mortality in untreated severe depression, ECT can be construed as a life-saving treatment in some cases.

ECT may also actually be safer in the elderly (compared to tricyclics) because it lacks cardiotoxicity. It is not without risk though (1:30 000 mortality compared to dental anaesthesia which has a 1:300 000 mortality). Cerebral systolic blood pressure rises to 200 mmHG during the fit and so vascular aneurysms may burst. Recent cerebrovascular accidents and myocardial infarctions are relative contraindications. Raised intracranial pressure is an absolute contraindication.

ECT has effects on memory formation causing a retrograde amnesia, a confused phase following the convulsion and a period of anterograde amnesia. Conventional wisdom suggests that these effects are minor and reversible, but some patients complain of losing larger portions of memory. On balance though, considering the potentially devastating effects of major depression, ECT seems a more than worthy treatment.

Self-assessment

MCQs

1 Lithium carbonate:
   a is mainly metabolised by the liver
   b interacts with non-steroidal anti-inflammatory drugs
   c is lipophilic
   d is most therapeutic when serum levels are greater than 3.0 mmol/l
   e sometimes causes hypothyroidism

2 The following drugs are tricyclic antidepressants:
   a phenelzine
   b dothiepin
   c tranylcypromine
   d sertraline
   e lofepramine

3 Chlorpromazine:
   a affects anticholinergic receptors
   b causes photosensitivity
   c is a butyrophenone
   d is an atypical antipsychotic
   e is regularly given intravenously

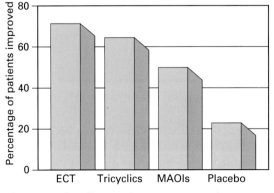

Fig. 15.4 The efficacy of ECT over 1 month.

Short answer questions

1 What are the side-effects of amitriptyline?
2 How does the pharmacology of lithium carbonate differ from the pharmacology of a serotonin re-uptake inhibitor?
3 Which foods and drugs must a patient taking phenelzine avoid?
4 What investigations need to be performed on a patient before and during lithium therapy?

Essay questions

1 Discuss the management of an anxious depressed patient with marked insomnia.
2 Discuss the long-term strategy for treating schizophrenia.

MCQ answers

1 a = F, b = T, c = F, d = F, e = T
2 a = F, b = T, c = F, d = F, e = T
3 a = T, b = T, c = F, d = F, e = F

Short answer questions — answers

1 The side effects of amitriptyline are those of a typical tricyclic antidepressant and can be recalled by remembering the different neurotransmitter systems involved: mainly anticholinergic (dry mouth, blurred vision are examples — you will need to list more), adrenergic (postural hypotension is an example), histaminergic (drowsiness) and non-specific effects such as lowering the epileptic threshold.
2 Lithium carbonate is an ion and is hydrophilic, excreted by the kidney and follows linear kinetics. SSRIs are generally lipophilic, are metabolised first by the liver and have complex kinetics.
3 Phenelzine is an irreversible monoamine oxidase inhibitor. Some of the foods and drugs to avoid are in the section above.
4 Full blood count, urea and electrolytes, serum creatinine, possibly creatinine clearance, thyroid function tests and ECG are the minimum necessary investigations.

Hints for the clinical examination

When taking the drug history remember:

- Finding out about the current drug history may yield vital clues to help you formulate a differential diagnosis.
- Ensure you ask about all kinds of medication including tablets, liquids and injections.
- Ensure you ask about overdoses; previous drugs that have worked well — these give a clue as to what might be a successful treatment in the future; dependency on prescribed medication; and previous experiences of ECT.

When you are with the examiners:

- Remember that management also includes family, social and psychological interventions as well as physical management.
- Use your knowledge of a few well-chosen examples from each drug category, but *do not guess drug dosages.*

Further reading and references

Texts

ASHTON H 1987 Brain systems, disorders and psychotropic drugs. Oxford Medical Publications, Oxford

BRADLEY P B, HIRSCH S 1980 The psychopharmacology and treatment of schizophrenia. Oxford University Press, Oxford

COOKSON J, CRAMMER J, HEINE B 1993 The Use of Drugs in Psychiatry, 4th edn. Gaskell, London

JOHNSON N 1988 Depression and mania: modern lithium therapy. IRL Press, Oxford

Papers

AGRES W S, ROSSITER E M, ARNOW B et al. 1992 Pharmacologic and cognitive behavioural treatment for bulimia nervosa: a controlled comparison. American Journal of Psychiatry 149: 82–87

ARONSON J K, REYNOLDS D J M 1992 ABC of monitoring drug therapy: lithium. British Medical Journal 305: 1273–6

ASHTON H, GOLDING J F 1989 Tranquillisers: prevalence, predictors and possible consequences. Data from a large United Kingdom survey. British Journal of Addiction 84: 541–546

CLINICAL PSYCHIATRY COMMITTEE 1965 Clinical trials of the treatment of depressive illness: report to the Medical Research Council. British Medical Journal i: 881–6

Elkin I, Shea T M, Watkins J T et al. 1989 National Institute of Mental Health Treatment of Depression, Collaborative Research Programme. General effectiveness of treatments. Archives of General Psychiatry 46: 971–982

Jacobson S J, Jones K, Johnson K et al. 1992 Prospective multicentre study of pregnancy outcome after lithium exposure during first trimerster. Lancet 339: 530–533

Kupfer D J, Frank E, Perel J M et al. 1992 Five-year outcome for maintenance therapies in recurrent depression. Archives of General Psychiatry 49: 769–773

Medical Research Council Drug Trials Subcommittee 1981 Continuation therapy with lithium and amitryptiline in unipolar depressive illness: a controlled clinical trial. Psychological Medicine 11: 409–16

Owens D G C et al. 1982 Spontaneous involuntary disorders of movement. Archives of General Psychiatry 47: 1023–1028

Rickels K, Schweizer E, Case G et al. 1990 Long-term therapeutic use of benzodiazepines. I: effects of abrupt discontinuation. Archives of General Psychiatry 47: 899–907

16

Psychiatry, ethics and the law

Most countries have mental health legislation to enable the state to provide care and treatment of severely mentally disordered individuals who, for one reason or another, refuse treatment. Such treatment is arranged for these individuals in the interests of their own health and the well-being of society as a whole. However, such legislation attracts controversy because it interferes with the autonomy of the individual. When is this kind of intervention justified?

Contents

The historical background

Some of the oldest written records document mental illness. It seems therefore that mental illness has probably always afflicted mankind. The Bible describes several people who could be construed as having mental illness, e.g. Saul had episodes of depression. Writing in the early years of the first millennium, Soranus of Ephesus described 'phrenitis', a disorder of thinking, which he distinguished from affective disorders such as mania and melancholia. Although it would be difficult to argue that Soranus's classification would be the same as ours, it seems very likely that he was dealing with a similar condition. In his form of mania he described grandiose delusions in which people saw themselves as gods, great orators, actors and even the centre of the universe.

Early forms of treatment

If mental illness has always existed, how did our ancestors treat it? Remember that they did not have recourse to antidepressants, antipsychotics or electroconvulsive therapy. If we look at written sources prior to the development of these effective treatments we can see that mental illness often lasted, in florid forms, for many years. In his authoritative textbooks Kraepelin described cases of psychotic depression that had lasted over 10 years. Victorian case records from Ticehurst House asylum document a person with depression who had nihilistic delusions that he had no stomach and therefore refused to eat. Over the course of his illness he was force fed with tube and funnel no less than 15 159 times using milk, egg yolk, beef tea, olive oil and brandy.

In the absence of effective treatment the methods available to eighteenth- and nineteenth-century society to deal with mentally ill people were usually either lock-and-key, with a varying standard of institutional care in prisons, houses of correction and private asylums or a negligent disregard, the sequel of which might be suicide or self-starvation. The main thrust of this 'treatment' was containment (Fig. 16.1).

Social attitudes towards mental illness

Mental illness was feared because of what the mentally ill might do and also because people themselves feared becoming mentally ill, for it was widely believed that there was 'no cure'.

At varying times and in different places throughout history, the mentally ill have been subjected to the consequences of society's beliefs about them (see 'Box' below). In some societies, the mentally ill

> 'The position regarding the so-called 'sacred disease' [epilepsy] is as follows: it seems to me to be no more divine and no more sacred than other disease, but like other affections it springs from natural causes.'
>
> 'Those who first connected this illness with demons and described it as sacred seem to me no more different from the conjurors, purificators, mountebanks and charlatans of our day, who pretend to great piety and superior knowledge. But such persons are merely concealing . . . their perplexity and their inability to afford any assistance . . . .'
>
> *Hippocrates*
> *Greek physician practising in Thrace, Thessaly and Macedonia, who lived between 470 and 370 BC. He formed a school of medicine on the island of Cos.*

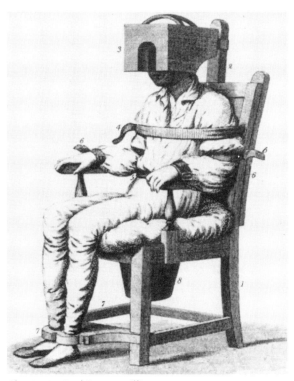

Fig. 16.1 Rush's tranquillizer.

have been seen as 'gifted' in some way, either as soothsayers or shamans, in other societies they have been seen as devil-possessed or witches. During the fifteenth and sixteenth centuries witches were routinely burnt or drowned throughout Europe. 100 000 women are thought to have died in this way. It is not known how many of these women were, in fact, mentally ill, but many of the signs of witchcraft that witch finders were trained to look for bear a decidedly close resemblance to psychotic symptoms and signs.

Incurability

The issue of 'incurability' has played a part in deciding the fate of the mentally ill throughout history. Roman physicians, as documented by Aretaeus, had the right not to treat 'incurables' and, as a result, the Roman mentally ill were largely warehoused in prisons. In Nazi Germany, psychiatrists were asked to divide their patients into two sorts, 'curable' and 'incurable'. The latter were gassed with carbon monoxide. At least 100 000 mentally ill and retarded people were killed in this way. This massacre of the mentally disordered was sanctioned by German law. Various films and books of the period, written by psychiatrists with Nazi sympathies, describe mentally ill people as 'life unworthy of life', and argued that their eradication was a blessing for them and a means of purifying the race.

Mental health law has also been used to enable sterilisation programmes for the mentally ill in many countries including the United States.

Humane treatment

Despite this appalling catalogue of tragedies in the name of law and society, we must also remember that history records many caring and thoughtful initiatives in providing care for the mentally ill. Forward thinking individuals like the Frenchman Pinel and the Englishman William Tuke revolutionised hospital care, transforming prisons into true asylums. Hospitals dedicated to the care of the mentally ill were in use in eighteenth-century York (The Retreat), fifteenth-century Spain (Hospital de los Locos), fourteenth-century London (Bethlem hospital), twelfth-century Baghdad (The House of

Grace), seventh-century Fez (The Moorish Asylum) and sixth-century Cologne (Monastery of Alexia). Private individuals, sensing the need for such care, have always founded small institutions or houses dedicated to the care of the mentally ill, for instance, Fabiola, a 'pious Roman lady' founded just such an institution in Rome in the fourth century AD.

We must not forget that we now possess effective treatments that can end episodes of mental illness and help prevent their return, thus dramatically improving the prognosis of affective disorders and schizophrenia.

The need for mental health legislation

There are perhaps six key points that we can learn from the short history above:

- Mental illness has occurred throughout history and we can predict from this that it will occur in the future of mankind as well and that there needs to be some provision to treat and prevent as much suffering as possible.
- Without treatment mental illness can persist for many months or even years, thereby blighting the life of the individual, their family and society.
- Some mental disorders rob their sufferers of insight and, consequently, they may fail to take treatment or care for themselves and, rarely, they may present a danger to others.
- There needs to be some means of giving adequate and justified treatment to patients who need treatment but are unable to make a clear judgement about their own mental state and health needs.
- In some countries in the past, mental health legislation has sometimes robbed the individual of their ability to reproduce and even lost them their lives. Legislation should be as reasonable, humane and open to scrutiny as possible.
- There needs to be a carefully monitored means of providing care under such legislation, i.e. there have to be adequate treatments together with trained people and regularly inspected places to administer that treatment properly.

Dangerousness

Apart from potential self-harm through self-neglect

or suicide, a particular concern of the media and society is the potential for dangerousness or harm to third parties. Such harm is rare, but may occur in a variety of mental disorders. Severely depressed people may see no future for themselves and others. Depressed mothers and fathers may kill themselves and their children in such circumstances. People with schizophrenia, in response to hallucinatory voices and suffering from persecutory delusions, may act on their psychotic symptoms to kill those they see as the root of their problems. Other individuals with personality disorders may enjoy harming others or setting fires, which may kill many people. One of the objectives of a mental state examination is, therefore, to assess the risk of harm to third parties.

An example of mental health legislation

In England, the 1983 Mental Health Act was drawn up to supersede and improve upon various Parliamentary Acts that dealt with the compulsory detention and treatment of the mentally ill, including amongst others the 1959 Mental Health Act, the Madhouse Act (1828) and the Lunacy Acts (1845 & 1890).

The current Mental Health Act has various sections which apply to people with a mental disorder, mental impairment or severe mental impairment. It does not apply to people without mental disorder or mental impairment. Thus the Act cannot be used to compel people who do not have mental disorder or impairment to have treatment. If they do have a mental disorder then treatment for that disorder can be given without consent if various provisions in the Act are fulfilled. There is a provision that any prolonged detention must be on the recommendation of two doctors and be applied for by either the next-of-kin or an approved social worker. This provision is to stop people being deprived of their liberty on the word of only one or two people. It has not been unknown for people to be incarcerated for fictitious mental disorders in order that relatives might gain their wealth. Furthermore the Act gives the right of appeal against detention. The appeal is heard by an independent tribunal appointed by a special commission, the Mental Health Commission. The tribunal usually has three people on it: a lawyer, a doctor and a lay person.

The Act has various sections that can be appropriate in varying circumstances. Section 5.4 of the Act allows a registered mental nurse to detain a mentally disordered in-patient against their will for 6 hours in order to allow time for a doctor to be found. Section 5.2 of the Act allows for any doctor, as a deputy of the responsible medical officer of the patient, to recommend the detention of a mentally disordered in-patient for 3 days or 72 hours.

Section 2 lasts for 28 days and allows for admission for assessment, during which time treatment can be given. Section 2 is applied for, usually by an approved social worker (one with Mental Health training), on the basis of recommendations by two doctors, one of whom should, ideally, be the patient's own doctor and one of whom should be approved under the Act as having special training in the recognition of mental illness. Section 3 lasts for 6 months and allows for admission for treatment. Section 3 requires the recommendations of a similar group of three people as section 2.

Other sections in the Act allow for police constables to remove people they suspect of having mental illness from a public place to a place of safety (section 136) or for the transfer of remand or convicted prisoners to psychiatric wards or secure hospitals.

Ethics and psychiatry

There are four main ethical principles behind a doctors' care for his or her patient:

- autonomy
- beneficence
- non-maleficence
- justice.

Autonomy literally means self-rule and would involve the patient's right to be informed about their health and using that information to make their own decision about whether or not to accept any particular treatment. *Beneficence* is a principle which, hopefully, lies behind the doctor's motives for helping the individual, i.e. a desire to do the best they can to help the patient. Behind it lies the idea that one ought to prevent or remove harm or evil and do or promote good. *Non-maleficence* would be a principle guiding the doctor to do no harm by his or her actions, i.e. not to cause damage to the patient by intervening or failing to intervene. *Justice* involves a sense of 'fair play' regarding, say, the appropriate and fair distribution of resources or ensuring that third parties come to no harm.

Doctors could use these principles to weigh up their actions or proposed actions to determine whether these were ethical or not. The ethical standards of a group, society or country are known as their *ethos*. Clearly the ethos of any particular group changes with the individuals in that group, the prevailing social beliefs and many other factors.

Groupwork: What would you do?

Form a group of colleagues together. Ask them to read and then discuss the brief psychiatric case histories that follow. Ask them to decide precisely what they would do and then ask them to justify their actions using the four ethical principles above. Try not to influence their discussion or their decisions, but record their deliberations. This experiment should give you an idea of that group's ethos. Repeat the experiment using a different group of people and record their deliberations. What do you think accounts for the differences in the ethos of different groups?

CASE HISTORY 1

You are a junior doctor in general medicine. Your consultant is consistently late for ward rounds. In the mornings he has a marked tremor and his breath continually smells of alcohol. He appears to be getting forgetful and is always mixing up his patients and their illnesses. Other more senior doctors on your team desperately try and cover for him. What do you do?

CASE HISTORY 2

You are a consultant psychiatrist. There is a change of government. The incoming party favour the policy of eugenics. Using the latest discovery (that major psychoses have a high genetic component) as justification, they pass a law to the effect that proven sufferers of psychotic illness must submit to sterilisation. You are asked to provide the

Home Office with a list of your patients. What do you do?

CASE HISTORY 3

You are an accident and emergency doctor. A 24-year-old man is brought in by his brother. Earlier that evening he had tried to hang himself after his marriage broke up. His brother cut him down and 'talked him round'. However, the patient had a change of heart later and took 24 tricyclic antidepressant tablets and 50 paracetamols to kill himself. His brother found out an hour later, by chance.

You see the patient, but before you can physically do anything the patient refuses to cooperate. You try and persuade him to cooperate, but he says he is a Law student and that any treatment by you without his consent is an assault. Unfortunately, he lapses into unconsciousness as you argue your case. What do you do?

CASE HISTORY 4

You are a consultant psychiatrist. An out-patient's family doctor asks you to visit her. She is aged 40. She is not eating and has not drunk anything since the day before. She says that there is nothing inside her and that she has no future. She wants to die and is lying immobile in a darkened room 'waiting for death'. You assess her and think that she has features of severe depression and ask her whether she will come in to hospital for treatment. She refuses your offer. What should you do? Is this in the patient's best interest?

CASE HISTORY 5

An 80-year-old lady is refusing to see her family doctor for routine screening which he is paid to do. He presses the point since his contract stipulates he should screen all elderly patients. She reluctantly agrees and in the course of a physical examination discovers she has a carcinoma of the vulva. He arranges an appointment with a gynaecologist with a view to surgical treatment. She refuses to comply. What can or should the family doctor do?

CASE HISTORY 6

You are a general practitioner. A 24-year-old man has been coming to see you 'in confidence' for puzzlingly trivial minor complaints. Now he tells you that he has been unsure of whether to tell you something he has been ashamed of all his life. Can you promise that you will treat it in absolute confidence?

You reassure him that you will treat his remarks confidentially. He tells you that he was sexually abused by his father until the age of 17. As a consequence he is worried about his own sexuality. However, whilst he is talking you realise with some discomfort that his 13-year-old brother is now being abused by the father. What do you do? Do you respect the confidentiality of the discussion or do you do something else?

CASE HISTORY 7

You are a general practitioner. A 21-year-old woman comes to see you about starting a family. Her husband is worried and has not accompanied her. His father died in his thirties of a movement disorder characterised by unintentional choreiform movements. His grandfather died in his fifties of a dementing illness and similar odd movements. Her husband is aged 23 and is asymptomatic. What would your advice be?

LEARNING POINTS

- Without treatment mental illness can persist for many months or even years.
- Some mental disorders rob their sufferers of insight and, consequently, they may fail to take treatment or care for themselves and, rarely, they may present a danger to others.
- There needs to be mental health legislation to enable the provision of treatment and prevention of as much suffering from mental illness as possible.

- Badly drafted or wrongly intentioned mental health legislation has in the past robbed the individual of their ability to reproduce and sometimes even their lives, so that such legislation should be as reasonable, humane and open to scrutiny as possible.
- Care given under such legislation needs to be carefully monitored to prevent abuses of power and to protect the rights of the individual.
- Ethical principles that should guide doctors include autonomy, beneficence, non-maleficence and justice.

Self-assessment

MCQs

1 Principles of ethical practice in medicine include:
   a ensuring payment for professional services
   b beneficence
   c upholding the autonomy of the individual
   d being a parent figure
   e justice

2 The English Mental Health Act (1983):
   a allows surgical operations to be given against the patient's will
   b contains an emergency section for assessment
   c provides for patients to be detained for up to three months without appeal
   d allows for compulsory psychosurgery against the patient's will
   e may compel patients to accept treatment for a mental disorder

MCQ answers

1 a = F, b = T, c = T, d = F, e = T
2 a = F, b = T, c = F, d = F, e = T

Explorations

Sources listed in the 'Further reading and reference' section will help you with the following:

Links with medical history

Psychiatry appears to be a discipline with an appallingly

bad catalogue of abuses of power, deception and folly. Is psychiatry different to other fields of medicine in this regard? Can you find any examples of ethical problems in the history of or current day practice in surgery, medicine or obstetrics and gynaecology? What are the key factors that allow such abuses or mistakes to occur? What principles can you identify that might prevent such mistakes occurring in the future? What was the Hippocratic oath and do we need a modern equivalent?

Links with forensic psychiatry

Forensic psychiatry concerns itself with the actions of the mentally disordered or retarded that bring them into conflict with the law. What psychiatric services are available to such people? What happens in criminal law to people who commit serious crimes but who are thought to have serious mental illness?

Further reading and references

Ethics, politics and psychiatry in literature

CHANG J 1991 Wild Swans. Harper Collins, London

Texts

BEAUCHAMP T L, CHILDRESS J F 1989 Principles of biomedical ethics, 3rd edn. Oxford University Press, Oxford

BLUGLASS R, BOWDEN P 1990 Principles and practice of forensic psychiatry. Churchill Livingstone, Edinburgh

DEPARTMENT OF HEALTH 1993 The Mental Health Act. Code of Practice. HMSO, London

DUIN N, SUTCLIFFE J 1992 A history of medicine. Simon & Schuster, London

FAULK M 1988 Basic forensic psychiatry. Blackwell, Oxford

GRAHAM L, PORTER R 1989 The hospital in history. Routledge, London

KRAEPELIN E 1913 In: Johnstone T (ed) Lectures on clinical psychiatry, 3rd edn. Baillière, Tindall & Cox, London

PORTER R 1987 A social history of madness. Weidenfeld & Nicholson, London

SCULL A (ed.) Madhouses, mad-doctors and madmen. The social history of psychiatry in the Victorian era. University of Pennsylvania Press, Pennsylvania

SEEDHOUSE D 1991 Liberating medicine. John Wiley & Sons, Chichester

Papers

MEYER-LINDENBURG J 1991 The holocaust and German psychiatry. British Journal of Psychiatry 159: 7–12

TURNER T 1989 Rich and mad in Victorian England. Psychological Medicine 19: 29–44

Index